The Mental Health Professional in Court

A Survival Guide

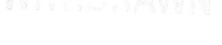

D1296888

0

The Mental Health Professional in Court

A Survival Guide

Thomas G. Gutheil, M.D.
Eric Y. Drogin, J.D., Ph.D.

Harvard Medical School
Boston, Massachusetts

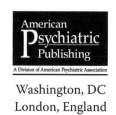

American Psychiatric Publishing
A Division of American Psychiatric Association

Washington, DC
London, England

If you would like to buy between 25 and 99 copies of this or any other American Psychiatric Publishing title, you are eligible for a 20% discount; please contact Customer Service at appi@psych.org or 800-368-5777. If you wish to buy 100 or more copies of the same title, please e-mail us at bulksales@psych.org for a price quote.

Copyright © 2013 American Psychiatric Association
ALL RIGHTS RESERVED

Manufactured in the United States of America on acid-free paper
16   15   14   13   12   5   4   3   2   1
First Edition

Typeset in Adobe's Optima and Warnock Pro

American Psychiatric Publishing,
a Division of American Psychiatric Association
1000 Wilson Boulevard
Arlington, VA 22209-3901
www.appi.org

Library of Congress Cataloging-in-Publication Data
Gutheil, Thomas G.
    The mental health professional in court : a survival guide / Thomas G. Gutheil, Eric Y. Drogin. — 1st ed.
       p. ; cm.
    Includes bibliographical references and index.
    ISBN 978-1-58562-438-6 (pbk. : alk. paper)
I. Drogin, Eric York. II. Title. [DNLM: 1. Expert Testimony—methods—United States. 2. Forensic Psychiatry—United States. W 740]
614'.15—dc23

                                                                  2012034984

British Library Cataloguing in Publication Data
A CIP record is available from the British Library.

To Shannon, always my inspiration—TGG

To LaurieAnn, the soul of patience with these writing projects—EYD

Contents

About the Authors

Thomas G. Gutheil, M.D., is Professor of Psychiatry and Cofounder of the Program in Psychiatry and the Law at the Massachusetts Mental Health Center and Department of Psychiatry, Beth Israel Deaconess Medical Center, Harvard Medical School, Boston, Massachusetts, and a former Distinguished Life Fellow of the American Psychiatric Association. He is the first professor of psychiatry in the history of Harvard Medical School to be board certified in both general and forensic psychiatry. A Past President of the American Academy of Psychiatry and Law, he is currently President of the International Academy of Law and Mental Health. Through more than 300 publications and international lectures and seminars, he has taught many clinicians about the interfaces between psychiatry and the law. He has received local and national teaching and writing awards and every major award in the forensic field.

Eric Y. Drogin, J.D., Ph.D., is a Fellow of the American Bar Foundation whose American Bar Association roles have included Chair of the Section of Science & Technology Law, Chair of the Behavioral and Neuroscience Law Committee, Chair of the Committee on the Rights & Responsibilities of Scientists, and Commissioner of the Commission on Mental & Physical Disability Law. A former President of the American Board of Forensic Psychology, he currently serves on the faculties of the Harvard Medical School and the Harvard Longwood Psychiatry Residency Training Program and is Editor-in-Chief of the *Journal of Psychiatry & Law*.

Acknowledgments

WE ARE indebted to members of the Program in Psychiatry and the Law (Massachusetts Mental Health Center and Department of Psychiatry, Beth Israel Deaconess Medical Center, Harvard Medical School) for years of stimulating dialogues that formed the substrate for this work, and especially to "Dr." James T. Hilliard, Esq., leading mental health attorney, for many years of advice and instruction and to Marilyn Berner, J.D., M.S.W., for helpful assistance with some sections. We also thank Robert E. Hales, M.D., M.B.A., for his meticulous reading of the manuscript and for his detailed, thoughtful, and supremely helpful critical suggestions and comments.

Disclosures: Dr. Gutheil has authored or co-authored about 300 publications, some of which generate income and some of whose content inescapably overlaps with this project. Dr. Drogin has no competing interests or conflicts to report.

Preface

How to Use This Book

Mental health professionals are among the many who are occasionally asked to go to court. It does not happen often, but when it does it is usually frightening, dismaying, or both. This book is designed to help you survive that experience. It surely will not turn any mental health practitioner into someone who *loves* to go to court—that goal is probably beyond the power of any book—but it may decrease the terror. Knowledge is not only power but also an antidote to unreasoning fear. Hence our purpose is to help you, the clinician-reader, become more knowledgeable about the settings, assumptions, personnel, issues, and techniques involved in going to court, with the aim of demystifying the legal process and reducing your anxiety about this inherently stressful experience.

Practically, this book is aimed at the professional whose knowledge about going to court is essentially limited to television and movies. At times, our review may seem a bit basic, but we have found in teaching audiences of our peers and colleagues that it is best to start from the most rudimentary position. This approach is the most inclusive and comprehensive and also may correct deeply embedded misperceptions and distortions of a sort typically introduced by standard media fare. Hollywood, after all, is not reality as we know it.

We begin with some introductory information about the basics of the legal process and its indigenous personnel and discuss some threshold issues, such as how to respond to a subpoena. Then we describe the type of witness you may be asked to be, how to work with your attorney, and how to prepare for a courtroom appearance. The final topics in this book include specific approaches to testifying on the witness stand and a review of the many roles that a mental health professional may play in courtroom proceedings. In these discussions, we have attempted to achieve as much verisimilitude as possible by drawing on examples from literally hundreds of actual cases and countless consultations with peers and colleagues on how to deal with the legal system. Along the way, you may also find some risk management advice to aid you in your likely goal of avoiding the courtroom altogether.

Three basic principles have shaped our approach to this book—a revised and expanded version of *The Psychiatrist in Court: A Survival Guide* (1998). First, it is written in an informal and at times even lighthearted tone—for easier mental access and for a soothing, supportive effect that is deliberately intended to allay your anxiety. Second, it consistently focuses on practical rather than theoretical issues. Third, its contents are brief enough so that you could read it all, if pressed, between the arrival of the subpoena and your pending appearance in court.

Because courtroom language is a dialect all its own, we have provided a glossary; legal technical terms in the text that are defined in more detail in the glossary appear in boldface type. Key points appear at the end of chapters by way of a basic summary. Two appendixes outline the legal system and provide recommended readings.

We hope that this book eases your journey through the legal system and serves as a useful navigational guide.

Thomas G. Gutheil, M.D.

Eric Y. Drogin, J.D., Ph.D.

CHAPTER 1

Introduction: "What? Me? Go to Court?"

FOR MOST mental health practitioners, the prospect of going to court—under any circumstances, at any time, for any reason—is about as welcome an idea as dentistry without anesthesia. Huddled around lunchroom tables in the hospital cafeteria, trembling clinicians share lurid tales of colleagues dragged into court and then, metaphorically, ritually disemboweled on the witness stand at the merciless orchestration of...the attorney.

The true facts are inescapable: citizens are flocking to court in ever-increasing numbers, for an ever-expanding set of reasons. Among those potential litigants are our patients or clients, who conceivably might (Heaven forbid!) sue us in a **malpractice** case. Even when not the direct focus of these festivities, nonforensic clinicians working in the trenches of patient or client care can be swept into the courtroom for a variety of reasons. If you are one of those so swept, we are confident you'll agree that some guidance would be useful—now.

The Mental Health Practitioner in Court

What could get you into court? We have already mentioned that a malpractice suit alleging problems with your care might do the trick, but there are other paths to the witness stand, some less widely known. For example, your patient or client might claim to have endured emotional **damages** from some event that lies entirely outside your purview. Because you are the treating clinician, your records and sometimes your courtroom **testimony** could be sought in connection with that damage claim.

More narrowly, a patient or client may assert emotional damages as only one part of a larger claim of injury. That claim, too, could drag you to court as the treating clinician. You also may be swept into a child custody battle involving someone you are treating, or into a discrimination lawsuit, or into a disability or worker's compensation claim. In summary, several roads lead to court, including many that have nothing to do with the quality of your care.

What Kind of Witness Are You?

The most common way for a mental health practitioner to end up in a courtroom is as a **fact witness** rather than as an **expert witness.** *Fact witnesses* testify about things that they themselves have done or about things that they have perceived through the senses: seen, heard directly (as opposed to hearsay), touched, tasted, or smelled. Fact witnesses also may, to a limited extent, testify about gestalts that typically emerge from these immediate observations, such as syndromes or diagnoses, and about immediate and actually occurring consequences, such as the drafting of a treatment plan or the application of a therapeutic intervention.

In contrast, *expert witnesses* may draw their own independent conclusions from data, including those gathered by other clinicians. They also may testify about abstractions, such as the "standard of psychiatric care" in a malpractice case. They may even render opinions about a patient whom they have never seen (e.g., in a malpractice case about a patient who committed suicide) or, in the case of the attorney's dreaded "hypothetical questions," about a patient who never even existed.

The role of the expert witness—one who actually seeks out opportunities to visit the courtroom as opposed to avoiding them—is covered extensively by other sources.[1]

Fact witnesses may be called on to play four roles in particular: 1) observer, 2) treater, 3) **plaintiff,** and 4) **defendant.** Following are some representative examples of each of these fact witness roles.

As an *observer* fact witness, you might be a bystander who was present by happenstance on an inpatient unit. Perhaps you saw a fight between someone else's patient and a nurse or some other interaction involving your own patient, a family member, and another doctor. As an observer, you are a "witness" in the narrowest, most literal sense because you just happened to observe (literally, to witness) a significant event. This event now brings you into the courtroom setting to report on what you saw, in the context of some litigation that really has nothing to do with you at all.

Another common role for the garden-variety mental health practitioner is that of the *treater* fact witness (more specifically, the nondefendant treater), who was caring for a patient either 1) before a claimed injury, typically to convey the patient's premorbid state; or 2) after a claimed injury, to determine the postinjury psychiatric condition in a manner relevant to alleged damages—in simplest terms, to let the court know if the patient has gotten better (or worse).

Third, you might be the *plaintiff* yourself. You might be suing someone else and might even have grounds to claim your own emotional damages. Informed by—but typically not emphasizing—your clinical knowledge, you might describe, strictly as a fact witness, your own symptoms and how they continue to affect your life.

Last, and most regrettably, you might be the *defendant* against whom the case has been brought. For example, in a malpractice case in which one of your patients alleges that you did not meet the applicable **standard of care,** you could state what you observed in this case and what you diagnosed; then, you could report what you did and your rationale for doing it.

To summarize, as a fact witness, you may provide direct observations, diagnoses, and descriptions of treatment—what you perceived and what you did yourself. Essentially, you are reporting narrowly on the results of your personal examination of the patient and drawing "conclusions," if any, that adhere closely to those firsthand observations (e.g., the patient's diagnosis and prognosis).

As reviewed in the next two sections, an ethical tension develops when a fact witness (in particular, a treater) is asked to perform the expert witness's role.

Treater Versus Expert

In general, these two roles—treater and expert—are considered incompatible because the clinical, legal, and ethical mandates are markedly different for each.[2] Because this subject is both important and often confusing, we summarize the critical differences between these two roles in this section, followed by a detailed analysis of how to avoid this and related pitfalls in the next section.

First, the expert does not enter into a traditional physician-patient or therapist-client relationship with the subject of the expert's examination (typically called an *examinee* or an *evaluee*). Second, the treater's job is to place the patient's welfare first—to help and to heal—whereas the expert's job is to teach and inform the judge or jury, by way of a report or testimony, regardless of whether the results help or harm the examinee. Indeed, from the expert's forensic perspective, the very need of the treater to help the patient constitutes a form of bias, through lack of the requisite objectivity and through investment in the outcome. Essentially, the treater's "client" is the patient; the expert's "client" is the retaining attorney or the court.

Further evidence of this dichotomy is found in the way that these distinct relationships are initiated. The expert is ethically obligated to warn the examinee that the material emerging from the expert's examination is not confidential and that results might be used in open court in ways that may or may not benefit the examinee. By contrast, in treatment, the clinician can usually promise **confidentiality,** barring a handful of technical exceptions and emergent circumstances.

Interestingly, psychologists adhering to standards promulgated by the American Psychological Association are ethically obliged to give the patient an elaborate protocol of warnings in the first session about the many possible forms of confidentiality breaches, as well as to tell the patient how to go about complaining regarding presumed ethical breaches.[3] Although we have seen no legal cases directly focused on this point, such a protocol would blur the distinction somewhat between clinical and forensic contexts because, arguably, the psychologists have given a quasi-forensic warning at the outset. In contrast, the ethics code of the American Psychiatric Association[4] does not require a similar protocol, although confidentiality and other requirements are explicitly identified.

The differences between treater and expert roles are even more readily discernible as the work of the treater begins in earnest. In mental health treatment—and especially in the treatment of trauma victims—it is important for the therapist to "believe" the patient's or client's story. The recipient of clinical services will not feel "joined" or understood without this form of acceptance. This technical recommendation to treaters extends, of course, far beyond trauma victims as a specific population. One might argue that all good psychotherapists attempt, through the process of empathy, to see the world through their patients' and clients' eyes. This deliberate credulousness (similar to the literary "willing suspension of disbelief") permits the empathic immersion in the patient's experience without which much of the therapist-patient rapport is unattainable, and successful psychotherapy is compromised. Similarly, such belief often functions as a kind of advocacy for the patient's view, which may aid in mastery of the traumatic experience.

The Treating Psychotherapist in Court: Some Common Pitfalls

In consultative experience, we consistently encounter an assortment of practical, conceptual, and ethical pitfalls (Table 1–1) that lead treating therapists directly into court—most often because these colleagues fail to understand the distinction between fact and expert witnesses. The nature of these pitfalls and the means of avoiding them are the subject of this section.

TABLE 1–1. COMMON COURTROOM PITFALLS

Subjective-objective distinction

Role conflict of interest

Economic bias

Difficulty in determining the standard of care

Hindsight bias

Goal-directed testimony and political activism

Why does this issue about fact and expert witnesses even arise? We have found that two types of attorneys most commonly precipitate this conflict: 1) those who simply do not understand the nature of the conflict and the irreconcilable roles of treater and expert; and 2) those who *may* understand this but who nonetheless wish to economize on expert fees by deliberately enticing the treater into assuming "double duty." Thus, in practical terms, treaters may be subjected to pressure from the attorney (or, on rare occasions, from the patient or client who hired the attorney) to adopt incompatible roles or may simply volunteer on their own to serve an expert function—out of ignorance and with a well-intentioned but ultimately counterproductive wish to advocate on behalf of the patient.

Subjective-Objective Distinction

An important aspect of the fact-expert dichotomy is that the fact witness's direct observations are overtly subjective, at least insofar as they are filtered through the treater's senses. In contrast, the expert strives for objectivity, which may include seeking out and endorsing views opposing those of the patient or discorroborating the patient's claims outright—two behaviors that would starkly ill accord with the treater's role.

The intentional credulousness of the treating therapist is, as previously mentioned, vital. If a patient said, "My mother is a terrible person," a competent therapist would never reply, "Oh, no, I've met her, and I think she's wonderful!" The therapist would grasp that the issue in question is the patient's subjective perception, not the mother as she objectively is or the therapist's equally subjective alternative view.

However, the same technically valuable credulousness becomes a ticking time bomb in the courtroom. Treaters are often in danger of failing to appreciate the degree to which their subjective immersion in the patient's experience constitutes an inescapable bias. Especially with trauma victims, therapists are in danger of confusing their therapeutic credulousness with actual knowledge of the external real event or trauma and then testifying on that basis.

For example, perhaps the individual being treated has an exaggerated and idiosyncratic reaction to what might be a minor trauma for the average person. Presented with a claim that the individual's life was forever changed by a billboard he or she observed or that a fall on the ice shattered forever his or her faith in a benign universe, the therapist accepts this (at least at first) as an emotionally valid description of an experience—an experience that does not necessarily mean entitlement to damages commensurate with those extreme feelings, even though the individual is unquestionably entitled to the therapist's compassion. The expert, in contrast, must bring such issues into perspective with reason, fairness, and reference to foreseeability.

Role Conflict of Interest

A second pitfall on the subjective-objective axis is the failure to perceive what amounts to a **conflict of interest** between therapist and expert roles. The best way to grasp this issue is to recall the physician's primary admonition, *primum non nocere*—"first, do no harm." The traditional interpretation of this principle is that the physician pledges to do only those things that will help the patient and, by implication, to refrain from all others that might be harmful. This admonition accords reasonably well—at least most of the time—with the role of fact witness.

Unfortunately, if pressed into the role of expert and honoring the new mandate of objectivity, the treating psychotherapist may well testify in ways that do not clearly help the patient or that may actually be harmful. Such an outcome necessarily occurs in a context in which the treater has neither warned the patient of this potential result nor disclosed the particular courtroom-oriented use to which the material exposed in therapy might be put. This situation poses an ethical bar to the treater functioning as expert. Therefore, all forensic examinations require a warning at the outset of the interview to inform the examinees of whatever limits of confidentiality or other ethical issues may apply to that interview and its later uses.

Economic Bias

Another potential pitfall in the treater's service as an expert flows from monetary considerations. Civil litigation usually involves damages. Technically speaking, *damages* are the amount of money considered by the decision maker to represent adequate compensation for the injury in question. In psychiatric malpractice cases, for example, this money is often earmarked to pay for the psychotherapy that the patient requires to overcome the emotional trauma the defendant has caused. Under those circumstances, the expert receives only a fee for having provided an evaluation and testimony and thus has no financial interest in the final outcome of the case; that is as it should be.

The treater, in contrast, has a direct financial incentive to be generous at best—or inflationary at worst—in defining the estimated damages because that money will go directly to the treater to fund the treatment. Although it is theoretically possible for a treater to remain free of bias under such circumstances, the appearance of a conflict of interest is damaging to the credibility of the plaintiff and hence to the strength of the case, if any.

Difficulty in Determining the Standard of Care

A central element in malpractice cases is the question of **negligence,** usually defined in terms of a failure to render care at the level of the average reasonable practitioner. Whether the care in question has met this standard is a legal question; depending on the **jurisdiction,** it may be determined by regional practice (the **"locality rule"**) or national practice as conveyed, for example, by peer-reviewed journals and the proceedings of national conferences. Focusing on the average maintains fundamental fairness; after all, it would be inappropriate to hold all practitioners to the level of the very best and then to assign fault for failing to meet that lofty standard.

The role of an expert in a typical malpractice case is to put forth an opinion as to whether the care delivered to the plaintiff did or did not meet the applicable standard of care. Most malpractice cases require experts to describe at some point how they became aware of the standard of care, especially if they practice in a different setting or devote most of their professional time to forensic evaluations. Enlightenment regarding this standard may come to the expert via, among other sources, 1) teaching or consultative experience; 2) organizational meetings, conferences, and seminars; or 3) peer review activities both for quality of care and for journal articles. In the eyes of the court, this knowledge base validates the expert's opinion.

Treaters are placed in an untenable situation when compelled to opine on the standard of care. They can scarcely be expected to depict the applicable standard as one higher than their own and are similarly unlikely to endorse a standard appreciably lower than the one they have devoted their professional careers to maintaining. This makes the treater's potential testimony a foregone conclusion—and foregone conclusions are anathema to the legal system's own standards of fairness (however much these may be seen as differing from our own). The treater should not be manipulated into insisting that "the way I do it is the right way, and other ways do not meet the standard of care." Such an egotistic, simplistic formulation would run seriously afoul of the pluralistic nature of modern psychiatry.

Hindsight Bias

Hindsight bias reflects the notion that retrospective vision is 20/20 because the events have already occurred.[5] When the psychotherapist is treating a patient or client whose previous treater was negligent, it is easy for the current treater to forget that he or she already knows the outcome (by virtue of hindsight) of the alleged negligence. However, knowing the outcome in the here and now does not necessarily mean that—from the "foresight" perspective of the previous treater—the outcome was foreseeable. The legal notion of foreseeability is essential to the finding of negligence: could—and thus should—the harm have been predicted under ordinary circumstances?

A particularly common pitfall is the subsequent treater's belief that his or her current knowledge of the patient or client is superior to that of all the previous treaters, even when the patient earlier had different symptoms or conditions. Again, the hindsight bias reveals itself: "I know what the outcome is, so I know retrospectively what others should have seen." Such a view is unfair to the previous treaters and slights the real and palpable data—much of it subjective and flowing from being in the actual room and observing the patient before one's eyes—to which a contemporary prior treater had access.

As it is with diagnosis, so it is with treatment. A subsequent treater must factor into the potential second-guessing of previous therapy the many uncertainties and ambiguities that may have been present in the past but that are now dimmed by the glare of hindsight and supplanted by the knowledge of actual outcomes.

Goal-Directed Testimony and Political Activism

The final pitfall represents a serious confusion of the political with the clinical and legal.

> A treating therapist serving as a plaintiff's expert in a sexual misconduct case stated, under **oath** in **deposition,** that she diagnoses posttraumatic stress disorder in all alleged victims of sexual misconduct, regardless of whether they meet the criteria, to ensure compensation for these patients.

Although one might understand the spirit of such a position, one also might reflect on how such an abuse of the diagnostic process may backfire, decreasing the credibility of this treater's testimony to the ultimate detriment of her patients.

The courtroom may be perceived as a hostile environment by many clinicians, but treating psychotherapists are increasingly called on to enter those precincts and give testimony. This review is intended to highlight common pitfalls for treaters entering into this "foreign territory." The major pitfalls addressed in this chapter include differences between fact and expert witnesses, conflicts of roles and interests, subjective and objective viewpoints, foresight and hindsight, and political contamination of the process. Armed with caveats derived from these discussions, the clinician may gain not only increased comfort—and appropriate caution—but also increased effectiveness as a witness in court.

• **Key Points**

- Witnesses may be fact or expert witnesses—the former being the focus of this book and of one's own compelled presence in court.
- Fact witnesses may be called as observers, as treaters, as plaintiffs, or as defendants.
- A court appearance is subject to many potential pitfalls, including role conflicts of interest, economic bias, difficulty in determining the appropriate standard of care, hindsight bias, and politically influenced testimony.

References

1. Gutheil TG: The Psychiatrist as Expert Witness, 2nd Edition. Washington, DC, American Psychiatric Publishing, 2009
2. Strasburger LH, Gutheil TG, Brodsky A: On wearing two hats: role conflict in serving as both psychotherapist and expert witness. Am J Psychiatry 154:448–456, 1997
3. American Psychological Association: Ethical principles of psychologists and code of conduct. Am Psychol 57:1060–1073, 2002
4. American Psychiatric Association: Principles of Medical Ethics With Annotations Especially Applicable to Psychiatry, 2010 Edition. Available at: http://www.psych.org/practice/ethics/resources-standards. Accessed July 16, 2012.
5. Yopchick JE, Kim NS: Hindsight bias and causal reasoning: a minimalist approach. Cogn Process 13:63–72, 2012

CHAPTER 2

"Why Is This Happening?"

It Is Not Your Fault

The mere fact that you have been sued does not mean that you did anything wrong. Even in a **malpractice** case—which means someone has alleged that you provided substandard care—there may be no one who believes that a problem was truly your "fault." As we will discuss, malpractice litigation occurs as the result of a complex net of circumstances that may have nothing to do with an actual failure on your part to do the right thing for a patient or client. Moreover, as noted in Chapter 1, "Introduction: 'What? Me? Go to Court?,'" many paths to the courtroom never intersect with your actual delivery of care at all.

It Is Not Even *About* You

Risk management workshops often urge the sued clinician to accept that a malpractice suit is not personal but rather just about insurance money. In our own experience, most of the many clinicians with whom we have consulted cannot really absorb such advice—let's face it: few of life's experiences will ever *feel* as personal as this. But there is more than a grain of truth in the objective view. Regardless of what sets it in motion, a lawsuit quickly transcends personal considerations to become a struggle within the legal system itself. To understand this better, let's review the psychology of litigation and some of its variants.

The Psychology of Litigation

Malpractice Litigation

Lawyers advertising on television (and there are a lot of them, aren't there?) often convey the idea that anyone who is disadvantaged in any way requires—no, *deserves*—an attorney who can achieve "big cash awards." A common phrase in these commercials is: "Injured? You may have a case!" This element of our current culture pervades the mass media[1] and forges a persistent link between "harm" of any kind and the lawsuit that surely must follow. But the link to care is overemphasized: your own experience surely will confirm that, at times, excellent care results in litigation, whereas clearly substandard care does not.

In the real world, usually malpractice litigation is initially driven by various emotions, alone or in combination, rather than by actual lapses in care per se. In fact, experience repeatedly indicates that malpractice suits result from a malignant synergy of a bad outcome—of any kind, for any reason—and bad feelings.

What are some of these bad feelings? Guilt is a very common one. When something bad happens to someone we love, we all wish we could have done more or done something sooner. *Survivor guilt* is a type of guilt commonly associated with bad outcomes: "They died, and I am still alive; why did I deserve this?"[2]

When a patient or client has a bad experience or even comes to a bad end, his or her relatives may feel this very guilt and deal with it by transferring it to us as treaters: "It wasn't *our* failure in some way to save or protect our loved one; it was the *doctor's* failure." Thus, litigation may serve in some cases to transfer guilt from the survivors. With this in mind, one can easily see that suicide—the worst outcome, leaving some of the worst feelings in its wake—would logically be the primary grounds for malpractice litigation among all mental health disciplines...and indeed, this is the case.

Another powerful litigation-driving emotion is rage, either in its direct form or in the form of outrage, even in minor forms. In some malpractice cases, the emotional wellspring was that the clinician tended not to return telephone calls. Other sources of outrage also exist:

> A patient in treatment for bipolar disorder committed suicide; the treating psychiatrist sent the widow a condolence card—an appropriate gesture—but enclosed in the same envelope the final bill. The ensuing malpractice suit

went up on appeals to the highest court in the state. Although the psychiatrist's adherence to the **standard of care** was ultimately validated, the true reason for the suit was clear.

Outrage may stem from a clinician's perceived rudeness or disrespect—even from simple use of a patient's first name, when that is felt as too familiar, condescending, or inappropriate. Yelling at patients or otherwise treating clients insensitively also may stimulate a litigation response. Arrogance and unavailability may do the same.

Grief is the normal human response to disappointment or loss.[3] The fact that grief is normal, however, does not make it welcome. Many equally human actions constitute attempts to avoid grief, including throwing oneself into activity. One such activity is litigation. Keeping busy with the various stages of the legal process may serve as a distraction from the bad outcome in question.

Surprise is a common trigger for litigation even when care has been fully appropriate. Numerous studies have documented how people with various forms of pain and distress may tolerate those experiences much better when they are warned to expect them. Surprise occasioned by a distressing experience makes most people scared and anxious, then angry, then potentially litigious.

Experiencing a betrayal of trust is another "bad feeling," a common source of which is the perception that the clinician is doing something not in the patient's or client's interest but in the interest of self-protection. Such "defensive practice"[4,5] is the most common form of alleged betrayal.

Imagine that a medical patient is discussing a planned procedure with a surgeon. At a certain point in the **informed consent** discussion, the surgeon states that "the law requires me to inform you of some things" and then begins a kind of rapid, monotonous chant: "There is a 30% chance...20% blah, blah...complications...side effects..." The patient's thought, meanwhile, is: "This is some kind of ritual, performed for himself, but he's not talking to me." Presumably, the patient's ability to retain any of this important information is extremely low. More damagingly, the patient's sense of the surgeon's self-serving behavior may be experienced later as betrayal.

Finally, feelings of abandonment represent a powerful stimulus to litigation. After a bad outcome, it is regrettably common for the clinician to back away from the persons treated or their relatives and to avoid contact, explanation, or even apology when such would clearly be appropriate. The patient or client may feel alone and left "out in the cold" with the bad outcome.

Actual experience indicates that these bad feelings play a significant role in whether a clinician is ultimately sued. Note again that only some of these feelings—and some parts of others—may be under the clinician's control. Regardless of the previously described principles, mental health professionals should get into the habit of calling their malpractice insurers when any "exposure" occurs; *exposures* are bad outcomes, threats of legal action, and even expressions of strong dissatisfaction with care. The insurer will have you speak to your underwriter to summarize the situation; take down your underwriter's name for reference. This step will not affect your coverage or premium, and useful advice may result. Most importantly, you will have given timely notice; lack of such timely notice may lead some insurers to refuse to cover you, should a suit develop.

Beyond lawsuits, the two other prominent occasions for going to court are complaints to the licensing board and ethics complaints.

Licensing Board Complaints

Board complaints differ in two important ways from malpractice litigation. First, the quantum of harm to the patient or client is secondary to the question of fitness to practice. In other words, the board's primary job is not to fix your mistakes—it is to make sure you are not someone who will make those mistakes again. Public protection is the board's stated mandate. Second, instead of addressing the issue of whatever compensation your malpractice insurer must pay pursuant to your policy, a board complaint threatens your license and thus your professional and personal livelihood.

You receive the complaint in the mail and a deadline to respond; if your reply resolves the issue, then that is the end of it. Things once taken for granted—like a full night's sleep and the ability to approach your mailbox without breaking into a cold sweat—take on a whole new meaning. If the board is not satisfied with your initial response, then the matter may proceed to a hearing.

Do not even consider responding to the complaint or attending a hearing without experienced legal counsel. You'll see more on this topic later.

The hearing, although not technically held in a "court," will be surrounded by all the trappings of one (including, often, attorneys on both sides), and the contents of this book will be just as relevant there. The proceedings are conducted before all or some of the members of the board—and surprisingly, it may be that none of them share your specific mental health discipline. You'll see more on this topic later as well.

Board complaints often tend to be based on matters the patient or client sees as too small to bring suit about—at least, yet—such as being treated in some disrespectful way. Perhaps the mental health practitioner has spoken in an insensitive, demeaning, or condescending manner or simply does not appear to have been listening. A patient or client may clearly sense—or, for that matter, have been informed by counsel—that these concerns are not what lawsuits are made of but concludes that complaining to the board may be a pathway to express this dissatisfaction, if only as a means to become "valued" or "noticed" at long last.

Please note that after the initial complaint, the patient or client, having served only as one who calls attention to a problem, "drops out" of the countertransferential equation at this juncture. The matter is thrashed out between the board and you.

Do not be misled by the supposedly small scale of the problem at the root of a seemingly "routine" board matter; all complaints should be taken very seriously indeed. Focused personal attention and in-depth legal counsel must inform your response.

Ethics Complaints

Ethics complaints are directed to the ethics committee of your professional society on the basis of a claim that you violated one or more of the canons defined in that guild's ethics code. Ethics issues may seem vague and variable to some, but ethics committees have a simplified role: ethics are what is dictated by the ethics code, pure and simple. After early exchanges related to the complaint, a hearing may occur, usually before the members of the committee. The roles of attorneys and hearing officers and the specific procedures for these hearings will vary considerably between organizations—and from those on display in board hearings—but many of these, including actual **testimony,** are clarified in this book.

Please note that all three of the actions described in this section—malpractice suits, licensing board complaints, and ethics complaints—may ultimately end up in the National Practitioner Data Bank if successful, serving as a cloud over your head for the future.[6]

Other Reasons for Going to Court

Some of the reasons for going to court, such as emotional injury or child custody fights, are noted later in this book. An additional pathway to court will involve criminal cases, whether these are against you or against a past or current patient or client of yours who is advancing a mental health defense (such as an insanity defense) for his or her alleged crime. Again, the testimony aspect of such cases will be aided by this book.

• Key Points

- The three major reasons for going to court are malpractice litigation, licensing board complaints, and ethics complaints; malpractice suits claim that we deviated from the standard of care, licensing complaints broadly address our fitness to practice or our merit as licensees, and ethics complaints assert that we committed a **violation** of some tenet of our profession's ethics code.

- Unless our particular insurer covers "administrative actions," only malpractice is covered; the other two ordinarily require out-of-pocket expenditures for one's own attorney and related costs.

- It is vitally important to contact your insurer at the first sign of serious dissatisfaction with care, of the threat of a lawsuit, or of a bad outcome.

References

1. Sahl J: Behind closed doors: shedding light on lawyer self-regulation—what lawyers do when nobody's watching. San Diego Law Review 48:447–478, 2011

2. López-Pérez R: Guilt and shame: an axiomatic analysis. Theory and Decision 69:569–586, 2010

3. Neimeyer RA, Burke LA, Mackay MM, et al: Grief therapy and the reconstruction of meaning: from principles to practice. J Contemp Psychother 40:73–83, 2010

4. Bishop TF, Federman AD, Keyhani S: Physician's views on defensive medicine: a national survey. Arch Intern Med 170:1081–1083, 2010

5. Hermer LD, Brody H: Defensive medicine, cost containment, and reform. J Gen Intern Med 25:470–473, 2010

6. Jesilow P, Ohlander J: The impact of the National Practitioner Data Bank on licensing actions by state medical licensing boards. J Health Hum Serv Adm 33:94–126, 2010

CHAPTER 3

"How Did I Get Here?"

The Path to Litigation

THE PSYCHOLOGICAL wellsprings of litigation were summarized in Chapter 2, "'Why Is This Happening?'" In this chapter, we summarize some of the common legal situations that trigger **malpractice** suits. The issue is also addressed extensively by several other sources.[1]

Suicide

For mental health clinicians of all disciplines, suicide is the most common basis for malpractice litigation. This makes perfect sense: reflecting on our paradigm of malpractice as something that stems from a combination of bad outcomes plus bad feelings, we can see that suicide is one of the worst human outcomes, one that is likely to leave some of the worst feelings in its wake in all the aforementioned categories of bad feelings. It is sobering to realize that clinicians may have limited means available to prevent suicide yet are often held to the standard of protecting the patient regardless.

In addition to primary treating clinicians, hospitals and their staffs may be held liable for suicides that occur during—or even some time after—inpatient hospitalization.

> A depressed patient was admitted. During the physical examination, his clothes were placed to one side and allegedly searched. This search appar-

ently missed the large-caliber handgun that the patient had brought into the hospital and used to shoot himself fatally. A suit for **negligence** was brought.

Boundary Violations and Sexual Misconduct

In the remote past, forbidden sexual relations with clients or patients were a dark secret in the helping professions, and by the mid-twentieth century, prominent **case law** still tended to recognize only actual sexual relations as the basis for suit. More recently, however, mental health professionals have had to track a complex and demanding array of boundary issues with patients and clients—requirements that have occupied the spotlight in a very serious but at times ambiguous fashion.[2]

> In a classic "slippery slope" model of increasing boundary transgressions, a therapist started calling the patient by her first name, then included some physical touch in the sessions; this extended to hugging, trips outside the office, restaurant dinners, home visits, and ultimately sexual relations. When the therapist refused to leave his wife, the patient sued successfully.

One way to look at professional boundaries in the context of mental health treatment is to regard them as constituting the "edges" of appropriate professional behavior. Unsurprisingly, what boards and courts will ultimately deem "appropriate" or "inappropriate" can wind up being highly dependent on context.[2] After all, some scholars have suggested that more than 400 named forms of psychotherapy exist, and one school's orthodoxy may be another's heresy.[2]

A useful paradigm for understanding this complex issue is to bear in mind the distinction between boundary "crossings" and boundary **"violations."**[3,4] *Boundary crossings* are minor deviations from formal clinical practice that neither harm nor exploit the client or patient. Examples might include offering a crying patient or client a tissue or catching by the arm an elderly patient or client who is about to fall; neither of these actions constitutes "psychotherapy" per se, but neither takes advantage of the person seeking services. The sharpness of this distinction can be complex, however.

> A patient repeatedly asked the therapist to call her by her first name; guided by instinct, the therapist politely but consistently refused. Later in the treatment, the patient acknowledged that had the therapist actually used her first name, she would have had to quit therapy because of the threat of implied intimacy.

Boundary violations, in contrast, are defined by the degree to which they harm the patient or client, typically by exploitation of sexual, financial, or dependent vulnerabilities. These actions not only form bases for malpractice litigation but also may represent ethics violations and grounds for board complaints. Examples might include requiring patients to perform menial services, such as cleaning the office or picking up the clinician's laundry; grossly and deliberately overcharging the patient; or engaging the patient in sexual relations. Several references address this topic in greater detail.[2–4]

Breaches of Confidentiality

In our experience, breaches of **confidentiality** usually flow from the "bad feeling" of surprise. The patient or client is taken aback to discover that disclosures to the clinician, offered in the strictest privacy, are now known by other parties. Such breaches can stem from ill-advised comments made within earshot of a **third party,** a letter or fax that arrives at the wrong destination, or some other release of private information without the knowledge or permission of the patient or client. Establishing some rules or practices with each patient is highly desirable.

> A therapist left a message on a patient's answering machine. The patient quit therapy and brought a complaint because the machine was in the family home, and others in the family, who had not been told that the patient was in treatment, now knew this fact, which the patient had wanted to keep secret.

Beyond the obvious need to exercise care when speaking, writing, e-mailing, or telephoning about clinical matters, understanding the role of surprise in such cases provides the best approach to help prevent the problem. We should enable those we treat to see and read everything that leaves our offices and to grant permission based on that knowledge. This approach avoids the surprise factor and provides an opportunity to discuss such matters in case of a concern.

Treatment Issues

The watchwords here are *too much treatment, too little treatment,* or the *wrong treatment*; concerns about side effects and claims of failure to obtain **informed consent** may play a role.[1] Although the problem may be clearer in the more concrete realm of psychopharmacology, psychotherapy, too, has pitfalls in this area. In addition to the boundary issues mentioned earlier, claims for needless prolongation of therapy, billing disputes, precipitous and inappropriate termination, and "false memory" cases[5–7] are the more common bases for claims.

• **Key Points**

- Common triggers for litigation include patient suicide, breaches of confidentiality, and boundary violations.
- An important distinction must be drawn between occasional mere boundary "crossings" and the sorts of boundary "violations" that can result in criminal or civil claims.
- Treatment issues of a more subtle nature that nonetheless may result in a visit to court include needless prolongation of therapy, poorly handled termination, and billing disputes.

References

1. Appelbaum PS, Gutheil TG: Clinical Handbook of Psychiatry and the Law, 4th Edition. Baltimore, MD, Lippincott Williams & Wilkins, 2007
2. Gutheil TG, Brodsky A: Preventing Boundary Violations in Clinical Practice. New York, Guilford, 2008
3. Gutheil TG, Gabbard GO: The concept of boundaries in clinical practice: theoretical and risk management dimensions. Am J Psychiatry 150:188–196, 1993
4. Nasrallah S, Maytal G: Patient-clinician boundaries in palliative care training: identifying and managing boundary crossings. J Pain Symptom Manage 41:263–264, 2011
5. Gutheil TG, Simon RI: Clinically based risk management principles for recovered memory cases. Psychiatr Serv 48:1403–1407, 1997
6. Simon RI, Gutheil TG: Ethical and clinical risk management principles in recovered memory cases: maintaining therapist neutrality, in Trauma and Memory: Clinical and Legal Controversies. Edited by Appelbaum PS, Uyehara LA, Elin MR. New York, Oxford University Press, 1997, pp 477–493
7. Raymaekers L, Smeets T, Peters MJ, et al: Autobiographical memory specificity among people with recovered memories of childhood sexual abuse. J Behav Ther Exp Psychiatry 41:338–344, 2010

CHAPTER 4

"What Is Motivating Everyone?"

You

You, of course, are trying to avoid any of the previously listed forms of **liability,** following the risk management approach mentioned at various points in this text (see Chapter 2, "'Why Is This Happening?'" and Chapter 3, "'How Did I Get Here?'"). If you should have the misfortune to become the target of a lawsuit, board complaint, or ethics complaint, you need to inform yourself as extensively as possible about what all the issues are, what to expect, and how to cope best with the proceedings. That is exactly what this book is all about.

The Plaintiff or Complainant

The patient or client who has turned on you is the **plaintiff** or complainant. When matters have progressed to a lawsuit, this person is called the *plaintiff,* and if a board complaint or ethics complaint becomes the avenue for seeking redress, this person is called the *complainant* (sometimes legal terms actually *do* make sense).

As clinicians, we can easily grasp how **malpractice** actions arise from the malignant synergy of a bad outcome and bad feelings, but that analysis, while valid, does not capture how the issue is viewed from the plaintiff's perspective. What plaintiffs want, according to surveys of that population, can be termed the *three R's:* recognition, remorse, and remedy (L. Crawford, personal communication, December 4, 2011) (Table 4–1).

TABLE 4–1.   WHAT PLAINTIFFS REALLY WANT: THE THREE R'S

Recognition	Acknowledgment that they were truly harmed
Remorse	The treater's actual and expressed regret for the harm
Remedy	Compensation for the harm and prevention of future harm

---

Recognition is related to the wish on the part of those allegedly injured— even by forces beyond the clinician's control—to have the treater acknowledge (or admit) that something bad actually happened: that the injury is real. The treater's natural human impulse to deny and defend turns out only to fuel the fires that result in litigation. Plaintiffs and complainants often have been heard to comment that "if only the doctor had admitted that he did something wrong and hurt me, I would not have sued."

Remorse speaks to the plaintiff's or complainant's wish that the treater both feel and express regret for the bad outcome in question. On occasion, the central component of this expressed regret is a formal apology. During the past decade in particular, a virtual science of the apology—too evolved and extensive to address here—has sprung up in relation to the legal and administrative management of clinical mishaps.[1,2]

Remedy is a twofold notion. First, it can refer to the plaintiff's or complainant's wish that steps be taken to prevent whatever went wrong this time from happening again; indeed, some—truthfully or not—offer this as the reason they brought the suit in the first place, espousing an altruistic wish to protect others similarly situated from the same bad result. Second, it can refer to the plaintiff's or complainant's desire to be compensated for what he or she has been forced to endure—what the legal system refers to as being "made whole."[3]

Each of the three R's usually calls for sensitivity and delicacy when dealing with allegedly injured patients and clients. The uneven distribution of such qualities, even among highly experienced psychotherapists, is something that should be acknowledged with all due candor. This is one of the many reasons that risk management advisers insist that negotiations should be handled by those whose professional role is to solve problems legally as opposed to clinically.

Do not even consider contacting a plaintiff or complainant on your own once a lawsuit, board complaint, or ethics complaint has been initiated. You will see more on this topic later.

Opposing (Plaintiff's) Counsel

One finer point of the psychology of litigation involves understanding that an attorney is not usually the first resort for a distressed patient or client. Most of these persons first seek to obtain a response from the treater. When that effort meets with resistance—including denial, stonewalling, avoidance, and unavailability—the allegedly injured party seeks outside help. As suggested in Chapter 2, lawyers' television commercials can provide considerable reinforcement and even initial stimulus to this decision by stressing the link between an injury and the "need" for litigation.

Opposing counsel is in a complex position in a malpractice case: there is no lawsuit until someone actually files it. Plaintiffs' attorneys essentially create a case from "scratch" in a very concrete sense because they typically must front most or all of the money for initial expenses and will collect a fee of their own only if they win the case.[4]

This means that opposing counsel should carefully assess the "winnability" of a potential lawsuit. Most ethical and competent attorneys undertake this analysis with all due diligence. Despite the common perception that the plaintiff's bar is possessed of a lottery mentality—"What the hell, I'll sue whether there seems to be a case or not…and I might win"—only the desperate and the bottom feeders have dedicated their legal careers to such practices.

Opposing Counsel's Expert

The opposing counsel's expert performs a critical function in the opposing counsel's attempts to evaluate the strength of the case against you. The attorney will never achieve the necessary depth of understanding concerning what transpired with patients and clients unless a mental health professional explains it. Moreover, some **jurisdictions** actually require an initial screening of malpractice matters by a professional sharing the same discipline as the **defendant,** and some also require an affidavit from that professional, stating that the case is likely to have "merit." Still other jurisdictions employ a panel or tribunal to perform this initial triaging function.[5] Although such mechanisms are intended to keep the courts free of trivial or "nuisance" suits, they do not always succeed in this laudable goal.

From your viewpoint as the defendant, the natural question is: "Why is this fellow practitioner attempting to destroy my profession…my career…my life?" In reality, your destruction is not the goal of these proceedings, which actually are intended, as in all civil suits, to provide compensation for losses experienced by the injured.

Our legal system requires an adversary model: two sides to every dispute. The plaintiff's side must be fairly and realistically represented, as must your defense. Experts for each side present their professionally informed views so that the **fact finder**—a judge or a jury—can weigh the opposing arguments and make a decision. Given how achingly personal this all feels, the cool and abstract workings of the courts doubtless provide cold comfort, but such proceedings are a reality of the clinician's professional life. Our aim in this text is to help you both avoid a negative outcome if possible and to be prepared should it occur.

Defense Counsel

Few things are as reassuring, amid all the anxieties of being sued, as having an experienced defense lawyer on your side. The mission of representing you in this process is taken extremely seriously by these attorneys, many of whom, through years spent in the trenches, know nearly as much about critical mental health practice issues as you do.

Unlike opposing counsel, counsel for the defense need not create a case, but he or she faces what can be an equally daunting prospect: taking on the case that fate has assigned, with the facts as inalterably fixed as the case may provide. Some cases—fortunately, a minority—are virtually indefensible. Most contain at least some positive elements that the lawyer representing you can muster in your defense.

Mental health professionals frequently wonder if they should retain, and pay out of pocket, their own personal attorney in addition to the one supplied by their malpractice carrier. Your insurer is your business partner and clearly would prefer to see you in the clear, but there are practical limits to how much your insurer will be willing to spend to support your cause.

As a general rule, this approach starts to become financially justifiable when a potential conflict arises—as, for example, when the same attorney represents both you and your hospital. At other times, sharing your concerns with your familiar personal attorney may alleviate some of your anxieties about the case in a manner that is privileged and cannot be used against you. If you find yourself in a serious personal clash with your insurer's attorney, the best solution may be to negotiate with your insurer for a change of counsel.

Defense Counsel's Expert

In the adversary system described earlier, defense counsel will be afforded an expert to present those aspects of the case that support your clinical decision making and to challenge or refute the claims of the other side. Some defendants, battered by the vagaries of the legal process, remark that they did not really understand the situation or regain a sense that they were actually reasonable clinicians until they heard their own side's expert testify. Your insurer's attorney can usually find excellent experts on his or her own, but you are free—and, indeed, typically encouraged—to make suggestions based on your knowledge of the field.

• **Key Points**

- The courtroom is full of many different persons, each with his or her own agenda based on some combination of professional obligations and personal goals.
- The individuals with the most powerful motivations will be plaintiffs and defendants as well as opposing and defense counsel and their respective experts.
- When you are interacting with plaintiffs, defendants, counsel, and experts, it is important to bear in mind how specific court-related goals will drive their behavior throughout the course of these legal proceedings.

References

1. Ho B, Liu E: Does sorry work? The impact of apology laws on medical malpractice. Journal of Risk Uncertainty 43:141–167, 2011
2. Regehr C, Gutheil TG: Apology, justice and trauma recovery. J Am Acad Psychiatry Law 30:425–430, 2002
3. Kian S: The path of the Constitution: the original system of remedies, how it changed, and how the court responded. New York University Law Review 87:132–206, 2012
4. Susser S: Contingency and referral fees for business disputes. Michigan Bar Journal 90:35–38, 2011
5. Norris DM: A medical malpractice tribunal experience. J Am Acad Psychiatry Law 35:286–289, 2007

CHAPTER 5

"Why Is This Taking So Long?"

Mechanisms of Delay

The anxiety and concern triggered by the news of an impending court appearance are instantaneous, regardless of whether you have been summoned for a **malpractice** case, a board complaint, or an ethics complaint. The actual proceedings, however, often appear to move with a speed that would make a glacier seem hasty and impulsive. Why is this so?

Although any claim directly affecting you appears to occupy your entire life horizon, your case is one of many—it has been said that suing one's neighbor has become America's second favorite indoor sport. But the numbers alone do not account for the scope of the delays.

Once they are filed or brought, all three proceedings—a malpractice case, a board complaint, or an ethics complaint—enter into a bureaucracy of some kind. The civil courts, the state licensing board, and the professional guild have a variety of built-in factors guaranteed to cast sand into the wheels of progress.[1]

Malpractice litigation requires some preliminary steps before anything substantive can happen. The case often must be tested for "merit" by some form of expert review, with interviews of parties and other forms of preliminary investigation amounting to what the legal system terms *discovery*.[2] Somewhere along the way, the case must be formally filed—along with an avalanche of other civil matters of every imaginable form.

Depositions (see Chapter 6, "'*Now* Do I Get My Say?'") require complex scheduling among several parties, you included. Should an actual **trial** eventually be necessary (see Chapter 9, "'Am I Going to Win This Thing?'"), attorneys will need to haggle over an even more complex orchestration of the presence of many persons, as well as the placement of your case into the court's existing **docket** of trials, some of them weeks long. In addition to these predictable factors, the attorneys, judges, and others may seek several postponements, called **continuances,** that reflect their commitment to other legal matters and any unanticipated problems within your case that need to be resolved before the trial can go forward.

Finally, life events may intrude, such as illnesses, personal emergencies, family crises, and previously scheduled vacations. Multiply the possibility of each of these by the maybe dozens of persons whose presence is deemed essential in the courtroom. A lapse of years between the initial claim and the actual trial is, unfortunately, not that unusual.

Although board complaints often have a slightly accelerated pace ("please respond to this complaint within 30 days"), the board may meet at only wide intervals, and its members are subject to the same potential delays that plague other civil proceedings. The board's thorough investigation of the details of the complaint may take a long time, and not all of its members may be available simultaneously. Many boards are understaffed, underfunded, and highly dependent on the uncertain participation of volunteer colleagues and lay members. The administrative law judges who often preside over board hearings seem to prefer to take a long time to think over and weigh their ultimate decisions.

Ethics committees of professional organizations face many of the same difficulties mentioned earlier, particularly the availability and consistency of administrative support, which are highly variable depending on the discipline and **jurisdiction** in question. Unlike courts and boards, the ethics committee may not have any prescribed deadlines for the processing of complaints or the scheduling of hearings, which can drag out the process even further.

Board and ethics complaints are not covered by malpractice insurance unless the policy contains specific reference to such proceedings. In any case, only a fool would enter either of these situations without retaining legal counsel.

Taking the Case Personally — or Not Seriously Enough

Taking the case personally or not seriously enough may interfere with your effective management of the stressful situation at hand. No amount of advice will fully erase the hurt feelings that come bundled with this process, but allowing a complaint to derail your life is probably overreaction in most cases. The events that triggered the claim are in the past and immutable. You have the assistance of capable counsel. You will be as well supported for the pending ordeal as possible.

Defense attorneys also frequently caution against not taking your case seriously enough. They mention this because encountering denial is as commonplace in their work as it is in yours. The mental health practitioners they try to defend frequently take the passive-avoidant position: "You're the attorney, so deal with it. I don't have time for this. I have patients to see." Although such behaviors would seem puzzlingly self-defeating, these clinicians are resistant to attending necessary meetings, providing relevant information, or performing needed searches for data. Viewed objectively, it should be obvious that this is a serious mistake.

The need to participate does not mean the need to call the attorney with each new passing thought—counsel, too, has other fish to fry. But participation does mean being responsive to the attorney's needs to master all elements of your case to defend you.

The Settlement Offer

The offer to settle a case has many alluring aspects. First and foremost, settling a case makes it go away.

Just like that.

Settlement bypasses the emotional trauma of a protracted proceeding, during which many clinicians feel that their entire lives are on hold. Settlement of a malpractice case does not constitute an admission of fault; many clinicians do not believe this point or just find it emotionally impossible to accept. The actual money is paid by one's insurer; sometimes even one's future premiums may be unaffected, or minimally so.[3]

For some clinicians, however, a settlement offer is seen as the siren's lure of the lazy attorney, the unsupportive insurer, or the vindictive patient or client: "They want me to admit I was wrong. They're trying to get me to 'confess.' I'll take this case to the Supreme Court, if I have to. I'll prove that I was right and that I didn't do anything wrong." Such colleagues often support this argument by noting that even small settlements are supposed to be reported to the National Practitioner Data Bank.

We can readily sympathize with this attitude, although ultimately it is not a useful posture to adopt. Transparently baseless cases are typically dismissed, often enough to ease clinicians' anxieties, and strong cases—even those with irrefutable evidentiary support—are usually settled because ultimately this is likely to be in everyone's interest. As a rule, only the ambiguous cases go (or at least should go) to trial. However, this truth offers cold comfort for a clinician on the hot seat.

The best perspective on this issue is a rational one, developed through searching discussion with your attorney. His or her knowledge extends beyond the letter of the law to issues such as how your case would play out in court, how your personal style and demeanor would affect a jury, how juries in your jurisdiction tend to decide, and which judges you should be glad—or concerned—to see on the bench. It's no accident that both of you wear the mantle of "counselor."

Bear in mind that the settlement offer is just one more move in the chess game of civil litigation. Together with your attorney, you should ponder the potential risks and benefits of this gambit as thoroughly and dispassionately as any other.

• **Key Points**

- Legal proceedings are subject to predictable and unexpected sources of delay; we cannot rely on them to unfold in an orderly manner that waits on our own personal and professional schedules.
- Clinicians must find a balance early between taking legal proceedings personally and not taking them seriously enough.
- Settlement is a potentially attractive notion that bears the advantages of finality and permanence; however, its options and consequences should be reviewed with counsel very closely before any formal offers are made or accepted.

References

1. Reda DS: The cost-and-delay narrative in civil justice reform: its fallacies and functions. Oregon Law Review 90:1085–1113, 2012
2. Lynch KJ: When staying discovery stays justice: analyzing motions to stay discovery when a motion to dismiss is pending. Wake Forest Law Review 47:71–112, 2012
3. Young GA, Clark JW: The good faith, bad faith, and ugly set-up of insurance claims. Florida Bar Journal 85:9–15, 2011

CHAPTER 6

"Now Do I Get My Say?"

Interrogatories, Depositions, and How to Survive Them

FOR MONTHS, even years, you've stood patiently by while the person you tried to help—and the lawyer he or she hired to attack you—have belittled your care, sullied your reputation, and drained your savings. All the while, you've kept your composure, never lashed out at anyone, and tried hard not to blame your patient or client for what may simply be a manifestation of his or her own illness. When is it *your* turn?

Interrogatories

Your first opportunity to inject your view of the case into the pretrial legal maelstrom is a set of queries called **interrogatories.** These questions are answered under **oath** and are designed to elicit certain basic facts about you and your practice.

One essential point must be made about interrogatories: do not even *think* of responding to them without defense counsel by your side. Although ultimately you will sign this document, the actual wording of your sworn responses will almost always require your attorney's careful crafting.

Bear in mind that if interrogatories appear abrupt, excessively accusatory, and unreasonably demanding, this just means that the standard procedures are being followed. Looking over this document for the first time can be almost as rattling an experience as when you received the initial complaint in the mail. Every book or article you've ever read about psychotherapy? Every continuing education seminar you've ever attended? Copies of your appointment calendar for the past 5 years? Are they joking?

The reason for opposing counsel's exercise in overkill is that any and all information can be useful in devising legal strategy—and that any and all deliberate or even inadvertent inaccuracies on your part can be transformed into powerful weapons against you during a **deposition** or **trial.** Interrogatories can be a classic example of what the legal professional calls "boilerplate," named long ago for unchangeable metal sheets of newspaper typesetting that looked like the panels once affixed to steam heaters.

Simply put, interrogatories always look like this. Don't view them as a sign that opposing counsel has singled you out for special punishment or that your care appears so shockingly substandard that its cause must be lurking in the recesses of a deficient and painstakingly exhumed professional education. Eventually, you'll get this paperwork filled out to defense counsel's satisfaction—and, in fact, your attorney may even advise that a legal basis exists for you to avoid answering some of the most unduly burdensome questions.

Depositions

As a **fact witness,** it is very likely that at some point in your career you will be called for a deposition. The purpose of this investigatory process is to aid each side in preparing for trial. The purpose of a deposition is to find out what you will be expected to say on the witness stand, to assess the strength of your potential **testimony,** to sample your demeanor and presence as a witness, and sometimes to preserve your testimony in the event of your unavailability through illness or a scheduling conflict. This chapter—among the most critical in this book—will prepare you for what to expect.

Mechanics of the Deposition

First, the physical setup of a typical deposition takes place at your office or conference room or at the office of one of the attorneys in the case. Location is largely a matter of scheduling and convenience. On some occasions, when the attorneys are from out of town, the office of a local law firm may be used for this purpose.

The cast of characters:

- You, the "deponent"—the one who answers under oath questions asked by the questioning attorney.

- Opposing counsel—counsel is sometimes alone and sometimes accompanied by a phalanx of attorneys for the **plaintiff** and for other parties to the case as well. These lawyers will typically question you in turn.
- Defense counsel—in hearings before a licensing board or an ethics committee, this person will likely be your privately retained attorney, unless, as noted in Chapter 5 ("'Why Is This Taking So Long?'"), your insurance policy covers administrative actions. Even if you have private counsel, the insurance company's lawyer also may be present and participating.
- The court reporter—in many ways, this is the most important participant. On occasion, other technicians will accompany the court reporter if the deposition is being preserved on video. The court reporter will be keeping a verbatim record with a stenographic machine, a computer, a sound recorder, or a strange-looking face mask that contains a microphone. Do not allow any of this to distract you.
- The complainant or plaintiff—in some cases, he or she will be sitting across the table from you for the entire deposition. You may be encountering this person for the first time since the complaint or lawsuit was filed. To the extent possible, do not allow this to distract you either.

In most cases, the attorneys begin by identifying themselves for the record and then stating whom they represent. They agree on certain ground rules, called *stipulations,* and then you are sworn in: an oath to tell the truth is administered to you by the court reporter as you raise your right hand. The language of this oath may vary among **jurisdictions,** but the intent is the same. The oath certifies sworn testimony under penalties of **perjury.**

After the oath, the questions can begin.

You usually will be asked if you wish to read and sign the deposition to check for errors. We strongly recommend that you do this because minor typographical errors and homophones can create serious misunderstandings (e.g., a leading journal recently apologized for a transcription error where the comment "it's an us-and-them situation" was transcribed "it's an S and M situation"). This becomes all the more important when considering that novice witnesses face the danger of "zoning out" from anxiety and not really perceiving each of the questions accurately.

Content of the Deposition

From the most basic perspective, a *deposition* is often described as an oral examination under oath, conducted as part of the discovery process whereby opposing counsel (usually) asks you questions to discover what you know and what your testimony at trial is likely to be. This straightforward portrayal, however, masks many pitfalls and misperceptions.

First, although this may seem like quibbling, the deposition is not the oral examination itself; instead, it is the *written record* of that oral examination, a fact that has a considerable effect on the intended uses of the deposition and how you should approach it. Most importantly, the information that is written down may be used later to challenge you, catch you in a contradiction, or impeach you.

One significant implication of this written record is the need to remain aware of its eventual audience. In the courtroom, you testify for the benefit of the judge—usually a former lawyer—and perhaps a jury, which is usually (although there are exceptions) a group of people with a high school education at best.

Because a deposition is a written record, this means that your true audience is the *court reporter*. This unexpected conclusion has certain implications for the manner in which you should answer questions.

To grasp this point more readily, picture yourself testifying at trial (please relax; this is just a mental exercise). In that context, you should be testifying—talking—in a friendly manner to the jury, attempting to seem relaxed (regardless of whether you feel it), and trying to use jargon-free, basic English without any complicated terms or subordinate clauses.

In contrast, in the deposition, you want to concentrate on several things. First, honoring the rule of austerity, there are five basic answers:

1. "Yes."
2. "No."
3. "I don't know."
4. "I don't recall."
5. A brief narrative.

Regarding the brief narrative, you want to make every effort to ensure that your answer cannot be quoted out of context. You do this by incorporating the question into the answer, despite how deadly dull this makes your answers sound (but remember, it is not the sound that matters; it is the court reporter's written record).

Thus, when someone asks, "Why did you consult the article by Smith and Chang prior to that psychotherapy session?," you could reply, "Smith and Chang outlined the best approach to…" but it is typically better to say, "I consulted the article by Smith and Chang prior to that psychotherapy session because it outlined the best approach to…"

The purpose of this strategy would be to keep opposing counsel from implying at trial—perhaps years later—that you endorsed the application of Smith and Chang's approach in *every* treatment situation, not just the specific one that presented itself at the outset of a particular session.

Put aside any fears about how pedantic and dry such responses must sound; you are creating a record for a specific purpose of preserving data, and you are avoiding creating a record that will fail to meet that purpose by being open to distortion.

If you disregard this advice, enter the deposition room, and start bantering and chatting and having a wonderful time conversing—under the deluded impression that you can charm opposing counsel into liking and "going easier" on you or that you can somehow tell how tough the questioning will be by opposing counsel's willingness to engage in social pleasantries—then you are not being sufficiently protective and careful of the development of the written record of your deposition. This lack of care may hurt you badly at trial.

To address this issue in another way, the language in a deposition should be precise, formal, austere, and self-sustaining for the specific question that was asked. In other words, the question should be incorporated so completely into the answer that even when the answer is read out of context, you technically would not need to know what the question was because you could infer or construct it from the answer you gave.

Preserving the Court Reporter's Sanity

Because the court reporter is your audience, it is important to understand how to keep him or her from experiencing a nervous breakdown (Table 6–1). Here are some tips:

TABLE 6–1.   TIPS FOR PRESERVING THE COURT REPORTER'S SANITY

Speak out loud.

Speak in turn.

Speak slower than usual.

Spell out technical terms.

Avoid banter.

Provide a business card.

- *Speak out loud.* Don't shrug, nod, shake your head, or grunt, because these gestures don't transcribe accurately. The reporter may even record these signs as constituting "no verbal response," which could make you appear to be withholding.
- *Speak in turn.* Don't overlap your answer with the question, even if the lawyer is asking a long, ponderous question to which you have long since figured out the answer. Stepping on the other person's inquiries drives the

court reporter crazy trying to write down what both speakers are saying. Wait for the other person to finish, and expect extension of the same courtesy to you. If your answer is interrupted, do not let this pass; state that you have not finished your answer, then finish it.

- *Speak slower than usual.* The court reporter has to document your answer correctly. Missing words can be critical. Getting back a deposition for review and finding it full of errors because you spoke too fast is annoying and a waste of time and money for everyone.
- *Spell out technical terms.* These include the names of drugs, diagnoses, and other bits of jargon unique to your field; this avoids wasted effort and is vastly appreciated by the court reporter.
- *Avoid banter.* The fact that the court reporter is your audience does not mean that he or she is your friend. Keep the relationship professional.
- *Provide a business card.* Offering the court reporter your business card before you are sworn is helpful if you have a somewhat unusual or often misspelled name and also encourages him or her to contact you if any questions arise about names or technical terms that you used, inaudible moments, and so forth. Some jurisdictions require that the court reporter see a picture identification card before starting.

Most depositions begin, after swearing-in and witness identification, with a set of instructions for you that are given by the deposing attorney. Pay attention to these, and try your best to follow them. The following is a real-life example of a witness not "getting it" when receiving an instruction during a deposition:

> QUESTION: . . . and likewise I'll wait for you to finish your answer before I ask my next question. Okay?
> ANSWER: Uh-huh.
> QUESTION: Also, if you give verbal answers, rather than nods or shrugs, the court reporter can take that down.
> ANSWER: (Witness moves head in an affirmative response.)

Note that this is one of several ways in which court reporters formally describe nonverbal responses. The purpose of these cumbersome locutions—"witness indicating," "witness moves head up and down," and "no verbal response"—is to ensure that ambiguous gestures are not credited as being substantive responses.

Some other useful methods for assisting the court reporter:

- If you don't understand the question, ask that it be repeated or read back as many times as you need for clarity.
- Turn to face the court reporter without worrying that the questioning attorney will feel you are rude.

- Speak slowly, distinctly, carefully, and in intact sentences.
- Take your time and rehearse your answer in your mind, looking for possible misunderstandings and distortions that might lie in a particular choice of words. You will surely find that your answers in this form will sound to you cumbersome, slow, affected, pompous, prolix, sententious, and perhaps even phony. None of that matters. You are trying to create a solid written record, not communicate to a jury.

Objections

At various points during your deposition, one of the attorneys may interrupt by stating for the record, "Objection!" In some, but not all, cases, the basis for this objection may be stated as well, couched in legal jargon such as "object to form," "lack of foundation," or "assumes facts not in **evidence.**" You should pause after each question anyway to take time to think and to allow for such objections to be made.

In general, objections are "just for the record"; that is, they do not preclude your answering but are designed to affect later **admissibility** into the trial process of the points under discussion.

Sometimes an objection is met with the question simply being withdrawn and a new one being posed in its place. At other times, once the attorneys have finished sparring over a question, you'll hear "you may answer." Unless your attorney actually instructs you *not* to answer, go ahead and reply.

You really do not need to worry about the technical bases for an objection because that is the attorney's problem, not yours. The following example is from a suicide **malpractice** case:

> WITNESS: I saw the patient run toward the window on the inpatient unit yelling, "I can't take it anymore!"
> PLAINTIFF'S COUNSEL: What was the patient trying to do?
> DEFENSE COUNSEL: Objection to form; calls for speculation. [The question seems to require the physician-witness to have read the patient's mind.]
> PLAINTIFF'S COUNSEL [attempting a remedy]: Based on your experience as a psychiatrist, did you entertain any concerns about the patient at that point?
> WITNESS: Yes.
> PLAINTIFF'S COUNSEL: What were they?
> WITNESS: I was afraid the patient was making a suicide attempt.

Under these circumstances, witnesses may appropriately state their own thoughts rather than trying to interpret someone else's.

You may hear at some point, "Objection—move to strike!" This remark may sound both startling and scary, but it is not your cue to duck under the table. Furthermore, it does not necessarily imply that your answer was untrue or that you violated some rule of deposition procedure. The attorney is merely flagging that part of the testimony for a future challenge to its admissibility as evidence in the proceedings. Alternatively, the attorney may believe that your answer was not responsive to the question asked, in which case the question will be either repeated or rephrased. The "motion" to strike that testimony may or may not be granted later by the judge. That is neither your problem nor your concern. Continue answering the questions.

Errors and Pitfalls

Clinicians commonly make certain types of errors the first time they are deposed. The first category of such errors is triggered by the erroneous assumption that a deposition is like a trial in front of a jury. Witnesses may think—wrongly—that they should focus on using the same casual, relaxed, and basic way of speaking that they would use in front of a jury, but a written record converts this into wasted effort. Witnesses playing to a phantom jury also may fail to remember that each answer needs to be able to stand alone in case it is quoted later out of context.

Alas, for simplicity, there is an important exception to the previously described rules: the videotaped deposition, which will be played for the jury in your absence if, for medical or scheduling reasons, you cannot travel; you are participating in another trial; or you are about to go on vacation. Videotaped depositions do not happen often, but when they do, they require a paradigm shift in your approach to answering questions. This form of deposition *is* the equivalent of a trial, in that the audience is no longer the court reporter but the jury, who will be seeing the entire give-and-take between you and the attorneys. In this situation, you should pretend that the camera is the jury. Look into the camera and speak to it using basic, juror-friendly, jargon-free language.

The second category of error is thinking that a deposition is somehow less *formal* than a trial. This often reflects a failure to recall that the deposition is an examination *under oath*. A deposition requires serious attention to truth and fact; you cannot just cheerfully make up information, "wing it," guess, or distort. Witnesses truly must "tell it like it is" because the looming issue of perjury is as explicit in this context as it is anywhere else.

A related pitfall involves assuming that this is "just a deposition," not a trial, and therefore you do not have to prepare as much—or prepare at all. Such an attitude is clearly a dangerous one, leaving you vulnerable to a damaging **cross-examination.** Your total mastery of the clinical case in question should be every bit as extensive as it would be on the eve of trial.

Leading attorneys have been quoted as saying that in a malpractice deposition, the primary goal of plaintiff's counsel is to get the clinician to concede **negligence.**[1] If you need any additional incentive as a **defendant** to avoid "deposition disasters"[2] by exercising vigilance and rigor in listening to questions and answering carefully, this is it.

The following article excerpt illustrates a physician's costly inattention during an actual deposition:

> During a predeposition conference, I asked both doctors to explain the patient's poor result. The neurosurgeon said: "When these discs protrude and compress down on the nerves, they often damage the nerves by compromising the circulation. You have to use very gentle retraction to move the nerves away to get at the disc material. But sometimes, even with the most gentle retraction, the nerves go into spasm. If we hadn't operated, she would have been a paraplegic. Her problems now are severe, but they had nothing to do with negligence. The damage was done to those nerves by the disc compression before we operated."
>
> His explanation was solid, and the neurosurgeon's demeanor made him a very strong witness. But at the deposition a few days later, the plaintiff's attorney asked, "Well, if you did such a good job, why is my client in this terrible condition?" Instead of his previous answer, the neurosurgeon replied, "Either Joey (the orthopedist) or I must have pulled too hard on her nerve roots."
>
> To this day, I don't know if that remark was a Freudian slip—or merely a slip of the tongue. But it was too late: That brief loss of concentration and an incredibly poor choice of words forced us to settle the case for $450,000.[3] (p. 158)

In addition, please note that one's professional colleagues, no matter how closely held in the bond of friendship, should be referred to by their professional titles: "Dr. Smith," not "Joey."

Common Attorney Deposition Tactics

Well-prepared witnesses—to say nothing of the poorly prepared!—should be aware of some common tactics that opposing counsel may use in deposing them (Table 6–2). These tactics are used not only to obtain that damaging admission of negligence but also to achieve other goals to your disadvantage.

Similar issues bear on depositions taken on behalf of your patients or clients. In this subsection, because your own goals will change in accordance with your different roles, the lawyer asking you questions will be described as the *examining attorney,* with the understanding that this is usually—but not always—a lawyer on the side of the case opposite to your own or to that of the person on whose behalf you are testifying.

"Let's have a conversation."

This disarming tactic essentially attempts to conceal that a formal and binding examination under oath is taking place. The examining attorney tries to relax

TABLE 6–2.   COMMON ATTORNEY DEPOSITION TACTICS
"Let's have a conversation"
"Changing up" the order
The "rhythm method" of witness control
An "end run" around objections
Deposition language
Getting you to "guess"
"Conversational" interjections
"Personal" questions
"Repetitive" questions

you with idle, nonthreatening exchanges—comments about the weather, re-marks about local sports teams, and so on. The seductive pull here is: "Let's just have ourselves a little chat, Doctor. I'm not going to take up a lot of your valuable time; I have only a few simple questions for you, so just relax." The novice deponent is in danger of being lulled into a posture of relaxed vigilance and casual, offhand responses to queries, forgetting that the written record may be used in later impeachment.

A related conversational pitfall is the *sotto voce* (literally, "beneath the voice") comment, a common element in many normal, everyday conversations. In a deposition, this type of remark is a dangerous example of "muttering for the record." The witness, struggling to decipher a Xerox copy of a progress note and becoming impatient, may mutter, "I can't make heads or tails of this," "I can't figure out *what* they were doing here," or "I can't make sense of this." In muttering so, however, the witness may later be characterized as impugning patient or client *care*, the delivery of which is recorded in the medical record. Rather than a mutter, a better "fully voiced" response would be: "I'm having some trouble reading this note; do have you a clearer copy or an original I could review?"

"Changing up" the order.

Depositions often proceed in a somewhat logical and hence predictable fash-ion, beginning with inquiry about your name, address, and social security number, and then exploring material from your credentials or curriculum vi-tae to get a sense of your background and training, as well as any special com-petence or experience you may have had relevant to the matter at hand.

Only then, usually, does the witness get to hear some questions that are directly related to the real reason everyone has gathered in the conference room. Minutes—even the better part of an hour—may go by before a single question is asked about the actual case. This is normal. Do not let this surprise or throw you.

Knowing that you have thought about your case and talked with your own lawyer, examining attorneys may try hard to keep you from telling a coherent, safe story. They may try to put you off balance by scrambling the order, beginning almost immediately with major questions. "What are all your observations in this case?" "After your patient shot himself on your doorstep, who was the first person you called?"

For many deponents, such queries have the startling feeling of an ambush and may rattle you—and indeed, they are specifically intended to do so. Your response, however, should not be impulsive, hasty, or flustered. If surprised in reality, you should buy "composure time" by saying something such as "I'd like to think about that for a moment." You should then pause and collect yourself, frame your response to contain the question, and respond, along the lines of: "Immediately upon discovering on my doorstep the tragic death of Mr. Jones, my first action was to…"

An extreme "scramble" can be seen in the following actual first question and answer from a case of therapist sexual misconduct [thanks to C. Bergstresser, Esq.]:

> *Question:* When was the first time you sodomized my client?
> *Answer:* I think it was in February.

The *"rhythm method"* of witness control.

Attorneys may try to set a pace or rhythm for the question—and, by invitation, your answers. Often, this approach is coupled with a "lulling series" of questions that psychologically prepare you to expect a certain response, after which the trap is sprung, as in the demonstrative mock example that follows:

> ATTORNEY (briskly): Doctor, did you beat this patient of yours with a club?
> PHYSICIAN: No.
> ATTORNEY (fast, almost on top of your answer): Did you stab him with a knife?
> PHYSICIAN (equally fast): No!
> ATTORNEY: Did you shoot him with a gun?
> PHYSICIAN: No!
> ATTORNEY: Did you give him medication?
> PHYSICIAN: No—wait—uh, I mean, yes, yes, I did.

As you see from the example, by encouraging you to "keep up with the flow," as it were, the examining attorney gets you moving to his or her rhythm, which may be faster than not only your natural rhythm but also your chance to think. As a result of this gambit, you don't have time to weigh your answers appropriately.

Resist the pressure to clip right along with the examining attorney; instead, sit there and think as long as you need to, until you have the answer organized in your mind, and then turn to the court reporter and give that answer.

Please bear in mind that later at trial, when your own attorney is asking you questions, getting into a rhythm with your questioner sometimes may be an effective method of conveying confidence or providing routine information. However, this approach probably should not be attempted by the beginner because it can easily sound awkward, false, or facetious.

An "end run" around objections.

Various attorneys participating in the deposition may be placing on record objections to certain questions; as noted earlier in this chapter, usually you will answer the question anyway unless specifically instructed by your own lawyer not to do so. At times, the examining attorney will attempt to "get into the back door" by making an end run around the objection—that is, by following up with a question only superficially different from the one just asked. Remember to pause for that moment and look at your attorney to see if he or she wants to object again or to give you an instruction.

Deposition language.

Persons watching a televised congressional hearing may well have come away with the following question (among others): "Why can't these ex-attorneys ask a decent question?" Apparently, going to law school does not automatically equip one with the ability make a coherent inquiry. Attorneys may appear incapable at times of asking a relevant, rational question in terms of organization, structure, and simple logic.

The following is an actual question that the examining attorney asked one of us during a deposition: "Was that explanation amplified in any way with any details as to what that sexual abuse was supposedly to consist of during that conversation?" Such a query calls for only one possible response: "Could you please rephrase that question?" or "I'm sorry, I didn't understand that." Don't even try to answer this kind of question; whatever your answer, there will be no way to tell what either of you meant.

Here is another "impossible question" asked by the examining attorney at an actual trial: "When he went, and had she, if she wanted to and were able, for the time being excluding all the restraints on her not to go, gone also, would he have brought you, meaning you and she, with him to the station?" The defense counsel replied, "Objection! That question should be taken out and shot."

Our experience has been that some attorneys think that they are effectively controlling witnesses by packing all possible subordinate clauses into the question, rendering it ultimately incomprehensible. In truth, this approach serves no one.

Witnesses themselves are not immune from a case of the "argle-bargles."
A real-life example follows:

> QUESTION: Have these symptoms [of posttraumatic stress disorder] been
> bolstered by research in biological abnormalities in the brain?
> ANSWER: Yes. This is a summary of some of the 1994 article by van der Kolk,
> "Biological Abnormalities in PTSD."
> QUESTION: Could you break that down into understandable—
> ANSWER: Yes, the psychophysiology. We've been talking a lot about that. As
> a clinician, that's the thing that you see. A lot of these other things are
> dependent upon blood studies, serum from spinal fluid, other kinds of
> research; methodology, much of it on Vietnam veterans and much of it
> carried on in Yale; in Connecticut, at the veterans hospital there; a lot
> of it being carried on at—in New York; and a lot of it carried on in Bos-
> ton. Okay. Extreme autonomic arousal reminiscent of the trauma. You
> know, I sort of described—I think I described that one. One that gets
> us here is what we call the neurotransmitters, and what we have
> found—there is an alarm system in the brain—and I'm going to show
> you that—but basically what happens is the noradrenergic system,
> which is noradrenaline that comes within the brain from the spinal
> cord, and epinephrine that you know about, comes from the gland on
> the kidney. I can't—I've got a blind spot here.

The true "blind spot" here is the witness's complete loss of perspective
taking. Apparently reading from some written material not identified in sufficient detail or without sufficient quotation marks to follow, the witness is
reading a bit, commenting a bit, editorializing a bit, tossing in the odd verbal
footnote, and addressing the attorneys a bit to remind them of previous points.
The result: an essentially incoherent record.

An additional difficulty is posed by questions that include double negatives. These questions come in a wide variety, but the common factor for the
deponent is that the same answer may be either accurate or the extreme *opposite* of accurate. In this regard, such questions resemble the "Have you
stopped beating your wife?" school of inquiry, in which an answer of either
"yes" or "no" is equally incriminating.

Here is an example, with emphasis added to highlight the double negatives:

> ATTORNEY (to defendant in sexual misconduct malpractice case): But you
> *never* had sex with him, *isn't* that correct?

To this query, "yes," "no," or even "maybe"—in fact, *especially* "maybe"—
would confuse this issue rather than clarifying it, as in that classic line "Yes,
we have no bananas." "Yes" in this context could mean "Yes, I did have sex" as
well as "No," that is, "You are correct, I did not." "No" could mean "I *did* have
sex, so no, you are *in*correct" or "Yes, I never did."

The only useful response would be either to request a rephrasing of the question or to take on the task of rephrasing the core point yourself: "It is correct to say I never had sex with him." Note also that your rephrased inclusion of the question effectively precludes later misunderstanding on the part of a jury if quoted out of context.

Getting you to "guess."

In normal conversation, your companion might ask, "Isn't Smith the chief executive officer of Widget Manufacturing?" You might not know at all or might not be sure, but to keep the conversation going, you might reply, "I think so, why?"; then the conversation would continue.

In casual conversation, no harm is occasioned by this sort of chat, even when you give an answer of which you were uncertain. However, if you guess at an answer during a deposition, you not only may delight the other side's attorney but also may have to eat your answer on cross-examination during trial.

Most often, the problem here is a basic human fear of looking foolish by not knowing something that you think you should know or that you think "they" think you should know. Here's the drill: even if you think that you *should* know, or that something is *usually* so, do not guess.

The following example illustrates why:

EXAMINING ATTORNEY: And when evaluating a patient, it would be customary to take a history, correct?
WITNESS: Yes.
DEPOSING ATTORNEY (confidently): Dr. Ramirez, your colleague, did in fact take a history from my client?
WITNESS (feeling the pressure to support the good doctor, and reasoning that she probably did it—hell, she must have done it): I believe so (although the witness doesn't actually know).

At trial, the witness can be made to look silly—or worse—when it transpires that the patient came into the clinic mute and catatonic, and the witness has inadvertently set the **standard of care** for his or her colleague to fail. "I don't know," "I am not sure," or "I am not clear on how that works" are perfectly good answers—when they're true. A similarly good answer is "I don't recall, but if you want to call my attention to something, I'll be glad to look at it." If the examining attorney shows you, then you get to see the source; if not, then the attorney looks bad, as though he or she were trying to conceal something.

"Conversational" interjections.

Consider the following example of deposition dialogue:

> EXAMINING ATTORNEY (appearing to set the stage for a review of the facts): So, you have this 24-year-old man…(attorney speaks in an "Are you with me?" tone, hesitates, and looks at witness as if for confirmation).
> WITNESS (tentatively, encouragingly, with rising inflection): R-i-i-i-ght.
> EXAMINING ATTORNEY: …who goes into the hospital…
> WITNESS (in a "keep talking" tone): R-i-i-i-ght.
> EXAMINING ATTORNEY: …and receives negligent treatment…
> WITNESS: R-i-i-i-ght.
> EXAMINING ATTORNEY (barely masking a smirk of triumph): …and is then discharged into the community…
> WITNESS (still oblivious to the prior slip): R-i-i-i-ght (and so on).

This sort of dialogue occurs countless times in informal settings; the storytellers check to see if their audience is with them, and the listeners send various socially sanctioned verbal and nonverbal signals. These signals include utterances such as "Right," "Wow," "You don't say," "Ayuh" (New Englanders only), "Uh-huh," "Yeah," a nod, and a head shake to convey ongoing attention and reassure speakers of continued interest.

In the preceding example, however, the written transcript is stripped of all this interpersonal and nonverbal "music" of tone and glance. The remaining bare words contain the witness's acknowledgment, almost in passing, that negligent treatment occurred, without the apparent realization that this wheel-greasing conversational interjection has essentially conceded the case to the other side. In such a situation, the witness should simply wait quietly until the entire question is out or respond, "I'm listening," until the time comes to give a fully descriptive answer.

"Personal" questions.

Examining attorneys may make personal inquiries as legitimate methods of discovery. Asking your date of birth, for example, provides not only your age but also some sense of career milestones, your experience in the field, or your seniority. Even questions on issues of a normally very private nature may have some arguably direct **relevance,** such as whether you are a recovering alcoholic, when the issue is your treatment of a patient with a similar condition.

Unfortunately, examining attorneys also may ask totally inappropriate and intrusive personal questions just to rattle you. Examples include the grounds for your recent divorce, your adolescent marijuana use, or the mental health history of your family members. The problem with such questions lies, in part, in the fact that no judge is present to rule on their relevance and thus to protect you.

Remember that you do not have to answer such questions if they genuinely have nothing to do with the case; indeed, a good answer to such an inquiry is,

"I choose not to answer that question, because I assert that my marital status has no effect on my testimony in this case."

If you choose not to answer, deposing attorneys may threaten to take the matter to a judge to compel disclosure. Fine; let them do so. In these situations, your own attorney can earn his or her pay as a representative and protector—in fact, you may even request a recess and attempt to call your personal attorney from the deposition to receive guidance. If indeed a judicial order is ultimately produced that compels testimony on a personal issue, then you will have to answer that question.

"Repetitive" questions.

Technically, an examining attorney is expected to ask each question once. One of the most commonly heard deposition refrains is, "Objection—asked and answered."

Although every lawyer in the room knows such an objection may ensue, examining attorneys will sometimes ask the same question, or minimally rephrased versions of that question, multiple times in an effort to see if you will answer differently. This difference could be used to impeach your credibility by the suggestion that you contradicted yourself. The examining attorney's underhanded efforts and your own attorney's strident objections may lead to some sparring in the deposition room, amplified by threats to go before a judge to resolve the matter. Stay out of the melee and wait patiently for the questioning to get back on track.

Where Should the Deposition Occur?

Most often, the attorneys involved negotiate where the deposition should occur, but sometimes your input will be solicited. Every possible venue has pros and cons.

The court reporter's company headquarters is the most neutral setting. This is optimal if the deposition is being handled by teleconference with out-of-town attorneys, because these firms usually have excellent setups for the audiovisual magic involved.

Meeting in one of the attorneys' offices is fine, although you are likely to feel somewhat out of your element. At least there will be no interrupting and distracting clinical calls because you will have arranged for coverage.

Your own office is, of course, home turf, but your professional library—not to mention your tastes in furnishing and decoration—are exposed and may be exploited in an attempt to rattle you. Perhaps the examining attorney will ask which of the dozen books on your shelf about suicide is the one with which you are most familiar and on which you rely the most. Do you consider this text "authoritative"? Can you describe its table of contents? The book lists "eight important ways to protect your client." The examining attorney wants to know if you can name them. "No? Can you at least name the first one?"

Reviewing and Signing

As noted earlier, once the deposition is concluded, you will typically be asked to review and then sign it. Despite our admiration for the skills and talents of almost every court reporter we have met, we strongly recommend that you take this task very seriously.

An errata sheet—a separate page on which you record the page and line of the error and your corrections—accompanies the deposition. This is not an invitation to alter your responses substantively, but you now can correct typographical errors and point out instances in which the content of your response was misconstrued altogether. Ask your own attorney to make sure you are addressing this task correctly. Such reviews also constitute an excellent learning experience because you can observe how you answered certain types of questions and then can consider how you might have answered better or at least differently.

Together with the signature page (on which your signature is usually notarized), the errata sheet is returned to the examining attorney and then distributed to the other lawyers as well. For convenience, some signature pages need not be notarized but are simply signed under pains and penalties of perjury.

A Model Instruction

The following dialogue is a model of an attorney's introduction to a deposition (all names in the example are fictitious). For completeness and thoroughness, you will be hard pressed to find its match (thanks to B. Baldinger, Esq.):

> EXAMINING ATTORNEY: Good morning Dr. Jones. My name is Jane Doe. I'm from Doe, Doe, and Roe, and I represent the plaintiff, Susan Green, in a case that's been brought up against you, as well as other defendants. I trust you've had an opportunity to review that complaint, and you are familiar with it.
>
> WITNESS: Certainly.
>
> EXAMINING ATTORNEY: I'm going to go through some basic instructions with you before we commence the deposition to make sure that you are clear about what the proceeding is all about. This is a deposition in which I, as well as other attorneys, have the opportunity to ask you questions pertaining to issues involved in this lawsuit. It is extremely important that you understand my question. If you don't understand my question, I'll ask that you tell me so; otherwise, we'll assume that

you understood my question and that your answer is responsive to it. Even though we're seated here in your lawyer's office, this is the same as though you were testifying in court.

WITNESS: Sure.

EXAMINING ATTORNEY: You've been sworn to tell the truth, the whole truth, and nothing but the truth, and that's what we all expect. On the one hand, if you do not know the answer to a question, it is perfectly acceptable to say that you do not know or do not recall. On the other hand, if you do have some information, I will ask that you give me what information you have that is responsive, to the best of your ability, to my questions. Do you understand these instructions?

WITNESS: I understand.

EXAMINING ATTORNEY: It is also very common for a witness or party to understand what it is that I'm asking and start to answer before I am finished. Please wait for me to finish asking my question completely before you begin to respond because the reporter can take down only one person speaking at a time.

WITNESS: Okay.

EXAMINING ATTORNEY: It's also very common to say uh-huh and nod your head. While here in the room we all understand, that is not translatable for the court reporter. You must say yes, no, and answer everything verbally. Do you understand that?

WITNESS: Yes.

EXAMINING ATTORNEY: It's fine if you use a gesture; just make sure you speak verbally. In the event that any of your attorneys or you hear an attorney in this room raise an objection to any of the questions, please do not answer my question. Please allow the attorneys the opportunity to put their objections on the record. You're instructed and directed to answer all of my questions unless your attorney instructs you otherwise. Do you understand that?

WITNESS: Yes.

EXAMINING ATTORNEY: Do you have any questions of this proceeding before we begin today?

WITNESS: No, I don't.

As a final point, remember that if the tension gets too high, or if you need a moment to regroup when you are feeling pressured, you can always take a break for water, for coffee, or to use the restroom; however, you cannot do so while a pending question is before you. Answer first, and then ask for the break. You are also permitted to ask for breaks to make time-sensitive calls or respond to pages. If you will have a planned interruption, such as a scheduled telephone call, it is courteous to inform the examining attorneys at the outset so that they can pace themselves accordingly.

It is also extremely important to ask for a break if you feel that you are mentally fatigued or that your concentration is slipping. Good deposition conduct requires an active and alert mental condition. Walk around, have coffee, splash cold water on your face—attempt to the best of your ability to attain full consciousness before resuming the deposition. A maxim often bandied about in these situations—applicable to lawyers and witnesses—is that if you are not tired and drained at the end of the deposition, you have not been paying close enough attention throughout.

Most competent attorneys can complete an adequate deposition, in a case of typical complexity, in just a few hours; however, don't count on this. A minority of examining attorneys may attempt to wear you down by needlessly prolonging your ordeal; if you are simply fatigued beyond comfort, ask your own lawyer if a follow-up meeting can be scheduled to complete your deposition at another time.

Depositions are serious and bruising business, but paying attention to the principles in this chapter will go far in cushioning the blows. Careful preparation both with your attorney and by yourself—an entirely acceptable practice in and of itself [4,5]—coupled with attentive concentration during the proceedings will ensure your survival.

• **Key Points**

- Interrogatories may seem at times to be intended for little more than harassment and confusion, but they must be taken seriously; counsel may be able to identify certain portions that can be answered in relatively brief fashion and perhaps even rejected with an appropriate explanation.
- Depositions are every bit as formal and consequential as trials or hearings and merit as much studied rehearsal and mental preparedness.
- Opposing counsel will attempt to apply several time-tested—but, fortunately, fairly predictable—tricks of the legal trade during depositions; these tricks can be overcome by witnesses who maintain proper levels of mental focus and professional integrity.

References

1. Fuchsberg A, Douglas PJ: Deposing the defendant doctor. Professional Negligence Law Reporter 7:193–194, 1992
2. Walvoord A: Coping with deposition disasters. Trial 48:30–33, 2012

3.   Griffith JL: Why defensible malpractice cases have to be settled. Med Econ 72:153–158, 1995
4.   Mester CC: Expert preparation. Trial 46:16–20, 2010
5.   Flowers RK: Witness preparation: regulating the profession's "dirty little secret." Hastings Constitutional Law Quarterly 38:1007–1027, 2011

CHAPTER 7

"Where Are We?"

The Foreign Territory
of the Courtroom

PRETEND FOR A MOMENT that your normally restful sleep is interrupted by a most disturbing dream. You find yourself standing on a high elevation in front of a crowd of people who are staring at you—perhaps, you reflect, because you're stark naked. Strangely attired persons bark what appear to be questions at you, about something that seems to be of great importance and meaning, but they are speaking a strange language. You can't determine what is going on and are thus helpless to respond.

To the clinician whose native turf is the quiet, familiar private practice office, the courtroom, like few other places on earth, presents the classic feelings of strangeness, helplessness, and nakedness typical of the worst nightmare. A trip to the witness stand combines all the primal fears: exposure, intimidation, helplessness, speaking in public, not knowing the rules, being made to look foolish, and so on.

To help you with these fears, let us propose a model for your first venture into court: treat it as though you were an American going to a mildly hostile, mildly intolerant, chauvinistic foreign country where they dress and speak quite differently—for example, France.

Your basic survival strategies would probably include studying important customs before your trip and becoming somewhat familiar with the language, especially some key phrases ("Pardonnez-moi, s'il vous plaît, où est le WC?"). You'll want to get acquainted with cultural assumptions and taboos and perhaps educate yourself on the proper dress code for various formal and informal situations. Although such anticipatory approaches would not solve all your problems, they would be likely to reduce them to manageable proportions. Such survival strategies also may make alighting in the foreign land of the courtroom less stressful—indeed, that is the very purpose of this book.

In this chapter, we discuss some of the basic cultural assumptions of the strange territory you are about to enter, with the goal of decreasing the strangeness of it all and of lowering your anxiety about traveling there. Additional aid will be found in the subsequent chapters and appendixes.

Fun With Your Tame Attorney

In foreign countries, you may not know which parts of the city are safe or which lovely forest glade may turn out to be quicksand. Surely a guide would be helpful. In the legal system, we call such guides *attorneys.*

In this section, *your attorney* refers to the lawyer you hired to represent you or to the one located and compensated for you by your insurance company. This individual can be of enormous assistance in helping you to find your way and to understand the strange linguistic turns given even to your own language. In today's litigious society, every mental health practitioner must have recourse to an attorney experienced in mental health law and attendant clinical issues.

The title of this section is meant to convey that clinicians will maintain the best possible handle on problematic situations that may arise at the medicolegal interface by developing a cordial relationship with the attorney on a regular basis—and well in advance of urgent need (hence *tame attorney*).

It is well worth your time and effort to canvass your professional colleagues for those attorneys who are solid citizens in this field and to spend a lunch or two meeting and discussing with such an attorney your career goals, type of practice, and so on. Mutual referrals may ensue. Inviting the attorney to address your professional society or practice group on a subject of current interest is an excellent icebreaker and a way to grant him or her access to potential business contacts.

The purpose of all this socializing is to move the attorney into the "professional acquaintance" category, so that when disaster strikes and you must reach out to someone, he or she will not be a stranger. If a medicolegal question arises before you have a chance to cultivate such a relationship, you will find that legal consultation services exist in connection with insurers, the American Psychiatric Association, and other professional groups. Ready access to such resources can be especially valuable, particularly to clinicians who routinely take on cases that involve high-risk populations and situations.

Finally, if you will forgive a personal bias, don't forget the value of touching base with a forensic mental health professional well versed in medicolegal issues.[1] This is not, of course, legal advice any more than it is psychotherapy, but the chances are greater that the resulting curbside consultation you receive will rest on a firm *clinical* foundation—a definite advantage.

Of course, attorneys can also be a source of grief as well as comfort, especially when mental health practitioners fail to take names and check affiliations from the outset of contact. An unsuspecting clinician may receive a call from a person identifying himself or herself as "the attorney on this case," only to find out later, after having conversed freely, that counsel is actually working on the *opposing* side of the case and that significantly inappropriate disclosure or other harm has occurred. Be alert to such fishing expeditions. If you have the slightest doubt about who the caller is and for whom they work, contact your own attorney before any further conversation.

Please bear in mind too that even a patient's or client's own attorney is not routinely or automatically entitled to a disclosure of confidential clinical information without proffering explicit written permission, a document that should be retained in your own files.

Do You Need to Retain Your "Personal" Attorney?

This is as good a time as any to revisit in detail a notion raised earlier in this book. A question that frequently arises when you are being sued for **malpractice** is whether you need a personal attorney over and above the one supplied by the insurance carrier if you are being sued in a malpractice action.

The short answer is typically "no" if you are a full-time private practitioner and typically "maybe" if you are a clinician who works in an institution or agency. The latter answer depends on whether the interests of your employer might diverge from those of your own. Do you really want the lawyer representing you *and* the hospital to have to weigh whether it is you *or* the hospital where you work that should wind up suffering the consequences of this lawsuit?

Retaining your own lawyer does not necessarily mean that he or she will be appearing in the courtroom to defend you. The insurer decides, for the most part, who that particular attorney will be. Engaging personal counsel is often primarily for personal consultation and reality testing throughout the legal process. Indeed, not all attorneys assigned to defend malpractice cases are able or willing to deal with the anxieties experienced during your first-ever malpractice case. With rare exceptions, conversations with personal counsel are not discoverable, so typically these cannot come back to bite you in court.

If you do retain your own attorney, be sure to notify the insurance carrier about this early on. If you work for a state or federal agency or institution, you may enjoy the protection of various tort claims laws, which can contain provisions that include caps on awards, immunities, or other limits to your personal **liability**.[2,3] However, if your own private attorney independently takes some legal actions that the agency's insurer views as prejudicing its defense of your case, this could compromise your legal relationship with your employer and complicate the protections you might otherwise enjoy. This issue should definitely be a part of your conversation with any lawyer who will represent you. Clear your actions with both sets of attorneys.

Some Notes on Malpractice

Psychiatrists have always placed low on the list of medical specialties being sued for malpractice, but, of course, low does not mean none. Historically, as noted earlier, cases in which a patient or client has committed or even attempted suicide have been the leading category of claims against mental health professionals of all disciplines. That primacy still exists.

Sexual misconduct cases and, lately, cases alleging harm from other boundary **violations** are on the rise as the second and third most common categories, respectively. Perhaps these will even change places before long— complaints for sexual matters have begun to diminish as those for nonsexual boundary violations continue to increase. Cases for breach of **confidentiality,** misdiagnosis and mistreatment, and harm to third parties are also among the most frequently occurring, with the precise order changing from year to year.

Predictably, budgetary considerations imposed by the advent of managed care have thrust an entire class of cases into new prominence, by some mechanism such as the following: an ordinary suicide case or negligent treatment case is complicated by the time allowed by insurance for hospitalization or treatment of the patient.[4]

For example, if a patient is discharged at the expiration of coverage and later commits suicide, the claim can be advanced that—had the insurance been greater or the practitioner willing to continue treatment—more treatment should have been undertaken, a longer stay might have been possible, and therefore the suicide might not have occurred. This kind of case adds a financial dimension to treatment that sets a disturbing tone for modern juries, who typically (and understandably) have their own axes to grind about financially imposed limitations to proper care. Such cases are so much on the upswing that some prominent mental health law attorneys have given up all other areas of practice and now make a good living solely on cases of disgruntled managed care customers who sue the agencies or the providers.

A more detailed exploration of current malpractice issues is beyond the scope of this book; suffice it to say that litigation is alive and well and may well be the reason for which you, the reader, find use for this text.

• Key Points

- Befriending and learning from the "tame" attorney is a prudent course of action and one to be pursued as early as possible before pending courtroom involvement.

- Forensically sophisticated fellow clinicians can be an important source of additional courtroom indoctrination and collegial support, as long as we remember to avoid delving into matters that could result in the need for additional **testimony** regarding newly shared information.

- The decision about whether to retain one's "own" attorney depends on several case-specific factors, and our eventual choices need to be shared with insurers and lawyers alike so that crucial protections are not heedlessly abandoned.

References

1. Bub B: Confidential litigation stress mentoring: thriving in the face of litigation. MD Advis 3:6–11, 2010
2. Cotet AM: The impact of noneconomic damages cap on health care delivery in hospitals. American Law and Economics Review 14:192–228, 2012
3. Salvi PA: Why medical malpractice caps are wrong. Northern Illinois University Law Review 26:553–562, 2006
4. Drogin EY, Meyer DJ: Psychiatric and psychological malpractice, in Handbook of Forensic Assessment: Psychological and Psychiatric Perspectives. Edited by Drogin EY, Dattilio FM, Sadoff RL, et al. Hoboken, NJ, Wiley, 2011, pp 543–570

CHAPTER 8

"Who Are All These People?"

You Can't Tell the Players Without a Score Card . . .

Although the exact roster will vary somewhat with the type of legal function in question, most basic roles remain the same.

First, the linchpin of the proceedings is a decision maker, called the **fact finder.** This may be a judge alone, a judge plus a jury, or—in some proceedings, such as a case before a medical licensing board in some states—an administrative law judge or magistrate.

Under ideal circumstances, the judge is a senior and skilled former attorney chosen, appointed, or (in some **jurisdictions**) elected because of superior intelligence and wisdom, exceptional knowledge of the law, incorruptible fairness, and objectivity. In other jurisdictions, the judge may be, as one Boston attorney put it, "a lawyer whose brother-in-law is the governor." Regardless, the judge rules the courtroom, and witnesses forget this primary rule at their peril. The physician may preside in the hospital, classroom, or private office, but here he or she is only a guest.

Regardless of the judge's failings or foibles (we recall one terrifying episode in which the judge underwent a paranoid decompensation while directly questioning a witness), the proceedings carry on. Serious errors must wait to be remedied at the **appeals** court level.

One of the most overtly "foreign" aspects of the judge's role is his or her confusing tendency to be identified in the second or third person in court-room parlance. For example, if an attorney is asking for some special consideration from the judge, he or she does not say, "If you would be so kind…." Instead, that request may be phrased in terms such as "May it please the Court…." The judge, too, uses the third person referring to himself or herself, as in "The Court finds that that **evidence** is inadmissible" rather than "*I find*…."

Judges are addressed directly as "Judge," "Judge Jones," or most often "Your Honor" and are thanked regularly; indeed, the proper response to most remarks that the judge may address to you is "Thank you, Your Honor," with few exceptions:

> JUDGE: Doctor, now that you have been sworn in, counsel will ask you some questions.
> WITNESS: Thank you, Your Honor.
> JUDGE: Also, please try to keep your voice up because the acoustics in this room are pretty bad.
> WITNESS: Thank you, Your Honor.
> JUDGE: Now, your name please for the record?
> WITNESS (carried away): Thank you, Your Honor.

Jurors are not addressed by name at all—at least, not by you. Look at them when you testify, smile at them, speak *as if* you are speaking to them, but otherwise leave them alone. If you think you're in trouble now, wait until someone sees you having even a casual conversation with a juror inside or outside the courthouse.

Jurors are historically intended to represent a cross-section of the broader community and to vote that community's collective conscience in the proceedings. Jurors are typically individuals with an approximately ninth-grade level of education, although some more affluent communities—for example, university towns—may field juries composed of mostly college graduates. This empirical fact places some weight on the witness's approach to language level and vocabulary, as we examine later in this chapter.

Almost always, at least two sets of attorneys are present, reflecting the workings of what the law accurately deems an "adversary" system. These persons are addressed as "Counselor," "Mr. Smith," or "Ms. Jones" and are thanked, if at all, only when they have done an appropriate personal favor for you, such as giving you time to refill your water glass or offering to rephrase a question for your better understanding.

The presence of multiple attorneys—a particularly common feature in **malpractice** suits—may confuse the novice witness. Let us say a patient is suing a therapist-counselor, a social worker, and a backup physician, all of whom practice at a hospital. The therapist, the social worker, the physician, and the hospital each may be represented by separate attorneys, under the theory that the interests of these parties may well be separate and may diverge, even though it is common practice for attorneys for an associated group of treaters to band together.

Do not be thrown off balance by the occasional archaism of one attorney referring to another as "my brother" or "my sister." This reference does not convey relatedness by blood; it is merely a traditional variant on "my colleague."

Commonly, but not always, a clerk of the court is situated near the judge. The clerk has a variety of functions, ranging from acting as the judge's gofer to serving as a legal researcher. Most often, clerks take notes, hand the judge relevant documents, check that witnesses are present, take telephone calls for the judge, manage the courtroom's increasingly high-technology recording and display apparatus, and mark exhibits—the latter involves identifying, with colored and numbered tags, the avalanche of documents or items of physical evidence that may be admitted as evidence in this proceeding.

A bailiff also may be present, usually attired in a uniform similar to that of a sheriff, police officer, or security guard. His or her job is to keep order and to prevent disgruntled witnesses, **plaintiffs,** or **defendants** from attacking anyone in court (in particular, think child custody). In some courts, the bailiff formally announces that court is in session and signals the imminent arrival of judge or jury. In others, the clerk may perform these functions.

The aforementioned court reporter (formerly called the stenographer) may be present to preserve a record of the proceedings, unless this role, too, is handled by the clerk.

The **oath** sworn by the witness to tell the truth may be administered by judge, clerk, bailiff, or court reporter, depending on codified rules and local custom. As an aside, the seriousness of this step—that is, the penalty of **perjury** for false statements under oath—is the same regardless. Recent authors of sociological studies on lying have reported its universality in human affairs, but the common conversational lie is a matter of personal moral outlook. The critical importance of truth telling in legal matters, however, alters profoundly the moral and legal context. *Perjury* is defined in the current context as lying in court while under oath. It is a serious crime that may itself be the subject of a **trial,** with serious penalties for a finding of guilt.

Every case has the parties, who are really the central players in these proceedings—the true reason that everyone else has gathered in court. In civil matters, you will find plaintiffs and defendants, whereas criminal trials have prosecutors and defendants (because the government is, in effect, the plaintiff). In administrative proceedings (e.g., against a clinician's license), the parties may be the clinician and the board of **licensure,** each represented by an attorney. In an ethics complaint, the clinician and the ethics committee of the relevant professional organization may or may not elect to retain counsel.

One final person—encountered less frequently than the others—is the **guardian ad litem** (GAL). The word *litem* is etymologically related to *litigation*. The GAL is usually an attorney (sometimes, a clinician or even a layperson) who completes a wide range of functions intended to aid the court in gathering information. These functions may include investigating a situation for the court as to whether a certain person, place, or situation actually exists where it is supposed to (e.g., is there such a person at a particular nursing home, and does he or she really need a guardian as claimed?); opposing the moving party in a proceeding to provide balance to the issue (such as challenging involuntary medication of an inpatient); or filling in to represent the interests of any party who otherwise would not have legal representation (e.g., representing a fetus in an abortion case). Because of direct judicial appointment in some cases, the GAL may be working outside the immediate adversary framework. From the witness's viewpoint, GALs generally should be regarded as if they were attorneys in the case until the witness is instructed otherwise.

Some Basic Rules

Like any social system, the courtroom has a set of basic rules and assumptions that are not always explained in detail. A working familiarity with these fundamentals will aid considerably in increasing the confidence, effectiveness, and survival of the novice witness.

The fundamental principle is the aforementioned notion of the adversary system. This reflects the basic axiom that legal truth is discerned by allowing the opposing sides to hammer away at each other—and that if the rules have been followed satisfactorily, then the prevailing party is justifiably the winner.

Those of us trained to use the scientific method as a primary truth-finding mechanism may find this arguably "might makes right" scenario figuratively and literally medieval. As the judge might say, "Your objection is duly noted"— however, mental health practitioners don't make the rules. That is why you have an attorney who knows the rules and frankly relishes the fight.

To grasp more clearly what the practical implications of this model may be, consider by way of contrast the way treatment planning is conducted in the clinical inpatient setting. If the treatment team consists of five members, experience shows that there will probably be five views of the patient and five opinions as to how that patient can best be treated. The team as a whole, however, must reach a consensus so that coherent treatment can proceed. This "wrangling of the pentalogue," as it were (i.e., a struggle among team members) must result in a best solution, even if it is a compromise. In the courtroom, however, the two sides battle in a zero-sum game—one winner, one loser—and only one party's true interests ultimately prevail.

Another implication of this model is the way in which ambivalence is treated. In real life, a given person may be ambivalent about a wish, even when the wish is one for compensation. In the court, no such ambivalence is expressed—one sues only to win. Arguments opposing your wish belong to the "other side." These arguments can lead to considerable uncertainty for the clinician testifying about the mental state of a patient or client, given the complexity, ambivalence, and multiply driven nature of the human condition. Such complexities do not fit easily into the Procrustean confines of the adversary system.

Another basic assumption that consultative experience shows to be problematic for the novice witness is the idea of the selective **admissibility** of evidence. In clinical planning, again, all input is desirable, although it may be accorded different weight. The views, observations, and interview data of even the most junior member of the team are sought and welcomed as part of the totality of clinical input to decision making. Half-recalled memories— of what the patient's second cousin may have said, as reported by the mother to the social work student and then passed on to the social worker who shared it with the team—may constitute valuable clinical data, despite the convoluted, hearsay-ridden trail by which it comes to the team's attention.

In contrast, an essential component of the perceived essential fairness of the legal system is the screening mechanism by which evidence makes it (or doesn't make it) into court. Fairness is seen as demanding exclusion, in the name of justice, of even some of the most concrete and compelling of evidence. We have observed time and time again that this exclusion is a particularly frustrating aspect of the proceedings for clinicians testifying in court. Despite taking an oath to tell "the whole truth," and despite the mental health practitioner's wish that the entirety of the patient's or client's story be told to the court to ensure full understanding, the extent of the information to which the witness can testify may be severely circumscribed[1]:

> A clinician was testifying in court for the second time about a case; the previous case had ended in a mistrial. Disclosing this fact, however, would have been deemed prejudicial to the jury. As a result, complex locutions such as "in previous sworn **testimony**" had to be agreed on so that attorneys and witnesses could refer to the earlier trial.

The need to adapt one's narrative impulses to the requirements of the legal system can place great strain on novice and experienced witnesses alike, especially those whose emotions have already been inflamed by the strangeness of the courtroom, the system's seemingly cursory disposal of the needs of persons with mental illness, and the occasionally abusive nature of interrogation by attorneys. Passionate feelings, however, do not justify attempting to force the court to hear what one believes it should.

In other words, answer all the questions, and then leave the stand. Judges are notoriously intolerant of anything that smacks of disruption or of preempting their authority, and the clinician who demands to be heard risks citation for contempt of court.[2]

This last issue brings us to another core assumption of the courtroom: its Socratic aspect.[3] Although there are many possible ways of telling a story, discussing a conflicted subject, or reaching the truth, the legal modus operandi is that of the question and answer (note, as a curiosity, that the Anglo-Saxon etymology of the word *answer* includes "swear to").

It may be useful to contrast this model with the one more familiar to the clinician: the case presentation or write-up. The organization of the latter follows a narrative flow organized into sections, which are essentially extended paragraphs: chief complaint, history of the present illness, psychiatric history, family history, and so on:

> The patient, John Smith, a 35-year-old Caucasian male, came to treatment with me on October 15, 2011, for depression and anxiety. I started him on a regimen of Prozac and psychotherapy, and he responded well....

Although there is occasionally room for narratives such as this in the courtroom setting, this crisp monologue might well be replaced by a far more extensive dialogue, governed by considerations that go beyond simply "getting the facts out there."

For one thing, the questions your attorney asks you cannot be "leading"; that is, the desired answer cannot be contained within the question ("You gave him 50 mg of Thorazine, did you not?").[4] On the other hand, similar-sounding questions may be used to define legally relevant points, leading to some rather strange-sounding exchanges:

> EXAMINING ATTORNEY: Doctor, are you familiar with an individual named John Smith? (Counsel and indeed everyone else in the courtroom may already know this, because Mr. Smith may have already testified to this effect, and the point may not be contested; it doesn't matter. This question is part of a background-supplying procedure known as "laying a foundation," on top of which future factual structures may be built.)
> WITNESS: Yes.
> EXAMINING ATTORNEY: Can you point him out to us?
> WITNESS: There (points).
> EXAMINING ATTORNEY: Let the record reflect that Dr. Jones has pointed to the plaintiff. (This locution, of course, deals with the fact that the witness's index finger is not visible on the written transcript.) Now Doctor, when did you first encounter Mr. Smith?

WITNESS: October 15, 2011.

EXAMINING ATTORNEY: And how did that come about? (This question is another redundancy, undisputed, already established—but not with this witness.)

WITNESS: He came in for a consultation.

EXAMINING ATTORNEY: And where did that take place? (Again, it probably did not take place in a telephone booth, but each element of the facts needs to be clearly established.)

WITNESS: In my office at Mercy Hospital.

EXAMINING ATTORNEY: When Mr. Smith came to consult you on October 15, 2011, what, if anything, did he tell you he had come for? (Although it is unlikely that Mr. Smith came for the consultation and said nothing—although sometimes that does happen in mental health contexts—the phrasing is couched so as not to make the assumption that something was said. Note also that queries such as "Why did he come to see you?" or "What did he come for?" are less proper because they leave unarticulated for the record how the physician would know. Reciprocally, the witness's answer also should address this point.)

WITNESS: He told me that he had been depressed for a number of weeks and that he was troubled by anxiety (rather than "depression and anxiety"; the physician, also, avoids appearing to know or to assume any ultimate truth beyond what the patient said).

EXAMINING ATTORNEY: And did you, in fact, undertake a consultation?

WITNESS: Yes, I did. (This last exchange, although perhaps logical and even redundant, is doubly necessary. First, the form of the question doesn't assume that a consultation automatically took place; maybe, somehow, it didn't. But more significantly and less obviously, the phrase "did you, in fact, undertake a consultation" in this context represents an offer of care such as might establish a clinician-patient relationship and the accompanying duty, relevant in a malpractice context, to render nonnegligent care.)

EXAMINING ATTORNEY: And what, if any, treatment did you administer? (The "if any" may sound to the novice witness like sarcasm or even like an implication that this physician would not treat a sick person who came for help; it is neither. Again, this phrasing avoids creating the assumption by means of the question that treatment was, in fact, administered.)

WITNESS: I started him on Prozac and psychotherapy.

EXAMINING ATTORNEY: And how long was Mr. Smith treating with you? (For reasons that remain totally unexplained, this awkward-sounding locution, "treating with," appears universally used by attorneys questioning treating clinicians.)

In later queries, the witness would be asked to define and explain both treatment modalities, to address the effects, and so on. Although it might be arguably faster to let the physician just spit out the story (and this is occasionally done with some **expert witnesses** when the judge is more permissive, more familiar with the witness, or just plain tired), the central method of obtaining testimony and building brick by brick the edifice of evidence remains the question and answer.

Subpoenas, Privilege, and Other Threshold Questions

Mental health professionals typically list among the scariest experiences of their careers the receipt of a **subpoena** in the mail or by hand from a constable or other official. Much of this fear appears to be based on what the subpoena is not (i.e., an arrest). Because the subpoena represents one of many pathways to the courtroom, we review it in this chapter.

Subpoenas are of two varieties: the regular *subpoena* and the *subpoena duces tecum.* The word *subpoena* means "under penalty"; you must appear in court under penalty of the law or be held in contempt of court. The phrase *duces tecum* from the Latin ("bring with you") means that when you appear, you must present to the court some relevant material, such as a patient's record or correspondence.[5]

In some cases, you will receive a fully expected subpoena for a court appearance that was planned some months ago and chosen from several dates you identified as the most convenient—and, in fact, you may be the one who requested the subpoena, as a means of establishing for your employer the necessity of your absence. In other cases, a subpoena may descend on you like a bolt from the blue.

From one perspective, the subpoena may be no big deal; attorneys have them on standard pads like prescription blanks and issue them as needed. However, although there may be steps you can take to avoid compliance, you cannot ignore a subpoena. Some form of response is required, and the best way to accomplish this task is to consult with counsel.

When you receive a truly unexpected subpoena, it may be helpful first to call the clerk of the court from which this document was issued and ask what it is about. The reason for this inquiry would be that it is often almost impossible to tell from the stew of jargon the subpoena contains just what the case is about. For example, you may know of a patient or client who died while under your care, but you may not recognize on the subpoena the name of the executor of that person's estate or be able to connect this name with the name of the individual on whose behalf your presence in court is being solicited.

Under various circumstances, and for several reasons, you may wish—or you may be advised by counsel—to have the subpoena legally cancelled; this action is called *quashing* the subpoena. Under other circumstances, your attorney, another potential party's attorney, or some other figure may attempt to quash the subpoena. Your presence may not really be necessary or even particularly desired, and, in fact, it may transpire that you were not even the mental health professional being sought in the first place. It also may be possible, when checking in with the clerk of the court, to open up negotiations for a less disruptive, later, or otherwise more convenient court appearance time than the one currently prescribed on the subpoena.

In considering the subpoena duces tecum, whereby material must be brought into the courtroom, keep in mind that this device merely gets some form of evidence into the courtroom; after that point, other considerations may apply. For example, the clinician who is asked by means of a subpoena duces tecum to bring a patient's medical record to court should not then immediately thrust the record into the first outstretched hand he or she encounters. Constraints may exist within the system to prevent **release** at all, or release to or beyond a certain extent, of the materials.

To grasp this issue, consider briefly the concept of **privilege.** Privilege is often contrasted—and confused—with **confidentiality.** The latter represents an ethical obligation of the clinician to keep matters identified during clinical work in "confidence" (i.e., from third parties), absent some specific permission to disclose it. *Privilege,* on the contrary, is a right belonging to patients or clients to bar material shared with clinicians from emerging in legal or quasi-legal settings, such as hearings, **depositions,** or trials.

The laws pertaining to privilege are complex and riddled with exceptions. Most nonlawyers cannot be expected to know or even understand them. As a result, as a practical matter, privilege decisions are usually a contest between attorneys and eventually resolved by the judge, as in the following example:

> A husband and wife were engaged in a child custody fight. During the divorce proceedings, the husband had sought psychiatric treatment to deal with the stresses of the dissolving marriage. The wife attempted to subpoena the husband's treatment records in the hopes of using the material to cast aspersions on his fitness for parenting. The husband tried to assert a therapist-patient privilege (available in some jurisdictions) to keep the records out of court. The judge ruled that she would review the records *in camera* (i.e., in private chambers off the record rather than in open court) to determine their **relevance.** The judge ultimately ruled that the records were not relevant, so they were, in fact, excluded.

Beyond the matter of privilege, other forces may affect the admissibility of clinical data. In some jurisdictions, for example, a court order rather than a mere subpoena is required to produce a medical record, especially when the information is being sought against the wishes of the patient or client in question.

One caution applies to both presentation of courtroom data and record keeping itself: the importance of distinguishing among sources of clinical data. In practice, this means being clear both in your mind and in the composition of your written notes where certain information comes from. For example, important distinctions may apply to data reported secondhand ("My mother said to me…"), thirdhand ("The nurse reported that the patient had said…"), and by direct observation ("The patient informed me that…").

It is also important to know and convey accurately what are clinical facts as opposed to legal ones. You intuitively know what a fact is, at least until you have to explain it in court. What complicates this situation is that the legal system uses the term *fact* to refer not only to the points on which the decision maker bases his or her conclusions but also to the conclusions themselves. This use of this term is why the judge, for instance, is referred to as a fact finder instead of equally viable labels such as decision maker, outcome determiner, or conclusion generator.

This can lead to some convoluted discussions and attendant procedural difficulties. For example, in a child custody battle in which child sexual abuse was claimed, an expert witness testified about how elements of the case were consistent, according to a forensic analysis, with that claim being false or unfounded. The judge interrupted with the comment that he had already found at an earlier stage in the proceedings, as a matter of *fact*, that the abuse had occurred. The witness expressed puzzlement at the alleged difference between legal and clinical uses of the term:

> WITNESS: It appears there is a difference between the legal and clinical views of the facts here, Your Honor.
> JUDGE: Let me ask it this way. If you assume the sexual abuse is true, does that alter your opinion in the case?
> WITNESS: (struggling to place this hypothetical question into conjunction with a clinical analysis of the case, which led to the opposite conclusion): Well, Your Honor (slowly and thoughtfully), if the abuse did occur, that would be a different case from the current one, so I guess my opinion would of course be different.
> JUDGE (triumphantly, as if just having proven the point): Right!

Some practitioners respond to this concern with the origins of information by using, or even overusing, the term *alleged*, as in "the patient alleges he has two brothers." It is probably more diplomatic to use the term only for sensitive material (e.g., "The patient alleges that he has a history of antisocial acts"). For routine recording purposes, "states," "reports," or even "says" convey the necessary source orientation, either in the record or on the witness stand.

Criminality and You

We certainly hope you never have to face criminal charges yourself, but there are two points to be made about this hope. In a growing minority of jurisdictions, sexual misconduct with a patient or client is a criminal offense and will be prosecuted as such—another among the many excellent reasons for refraining from such conduct.

Perhaps one of your patients or clients is involved in a criminal matter, with your testimony being sought to shed light on possibly relevant mental health aspects of the case.

Our consultative experience suggests that novice witnesses face two major pitfalls in these situations. First, as clinicians, we have a natural wish to help or protect our clients or patients; that's why we're in the field. However laudable they are, such intentions can clash with the legal system's need to focus on "just the facts." For the most part, all you know beyond your direct observations is what your patient or client actually told you. The goal of your testimony is to tell the truth factually—no more, no less.

The second major pitfall actually derives from the first one. Because we try to see the world from the patient's view, we often develop an erroneous sense or presumption that we "know" what actually happened outside the office because we saw it in our mind's eye. Things we think could not have happened may have happened nonetheless. We do no favors for our patients or clients, or for the legal system in which they've become ensnared, by speculating about the unseen.

• Key Points

- The identities, obligations, and behavioral quirks of judges, attorneys, clerks, and other courtroom personnel should be studied, understood, and accommodated to the best of our abilities, regardless of our particular reasons for being present during legal proceedings.
- Mental health professionals dedicate themselves to gaining as much information as possible to assist patients and clients and thus must remain on guard to avoid becoming confused and frustrated by the legal system's selective admissibility of certain types of data into evidence.

- Motivated by a desire to help and distracted by a penchant for creative speculation, we must nonetheless be aware of and scrupulously abide by the "just the facts" approach of most legal questioning.

References

1. Gutheil TG, Hauser MJ, White MS, et al: The "whole truth" vs. "the admissible truth": an ethics dilemma for expert witnesses. J Am Acad Psychiatry Law 31:422–427, 2003
2. Leal DM: Why there is disobedience of court orders: contempt of court and neuroeconomics. Quinnipiac Law Review 26:1015–1068, 2008
3. Dye DJ: Debunking the Socratic method? Not so fast, my friend! Phoenix Law Review 3:351–363, 2010
4. Brar J: Friend or foe? Responsible third parties and leading questions. Baylor Law Review 60:261–291, 2008
5. Buchanan JD: Subpoenas duces tecum vs. HIPAA: which wins? Florida Bar Journal 79:39–44, 2005

CHAPTER 9

"Am I Going to Win This Thing?"

The Trial Itself

FOR MOST clinicians, **trials** hold a terror driven in varying degrees by movies, television, and the awesome power of our own fantasies. Yet some knowledge and preparation can go a long way toward allaying some of the more gratuitous fears. Remember that the witnessing itself—the observations you made or treatment you provided—has already happened and is in the past. The testifying that now lies ahead is a kind of teaching to laypersons (judge and jury) about what you saw and did. As with other "tough audiences"—uninterested students, resistant patients—the setting is adversarial, but its challenges are not insurmountable, and at least one attorney in the room is on your side.

Some of the techniques and concepts that you have already learned for **depositions** will aid you in facing the stresses of trial itself. Some approaches will have to be altered or modified to fit the new context. In this chapter, we aim to prepare you for your appearance at trial. Bear in mind that in *this* context your designated role is a **fact witness** who knows certain information considered relevant to the case at hand. As a result of this specific function, you will be spared the necessity of defending your credentials and conclusions in the same manner as would the **expert witness** in court. First, some background material is in order.

A Nervous Trot Through the Law

Although one approach might be to walk you through the process of a case, the "gait" in the heading of this section seemed more suited to the affective context. The following discussions outline the legal system in brief and then trot you through the legal stages of the **malpractice** suit brought against you (for illustrative purposes only, please rest assured). Note also that some of the discussions found within this chapter constitute something of a review of issues examined earlier and that Appendix I outlines the legal system as a whole. First, we define some terms:

Statutory law is enacted by state and federal legislatures to provide a forewarning of penalties and obligations for all citizens. Thus, if your patient is charged with grand larceny, the definition and penalties for this **violation** of the **statutes** are written down and used by the criminal justice system. Statutory law may contain material relevant to civil actions as well, such as the criteria for an expert witness, standards of proof, and definitions of **negligence.**

Common law is the law of specific cases and **precedents,** decided by judges with reference to existing statutes and built up over time, with occasional changes and emendations.[1] For example, the *Tarasoff* case in California altered the common law by creating a new form of a duty of therapists to protect third parties from a patient's violent acts. Depending on whether cases have transpired on relevant topics, common law may or may not impinge on your participation in a court case. Your lawyer is your guide here.

The criminal justice system is somewhat familiar to most practitioners from television and film, where the various stages are often lingered over in loving detail by filmmakers to enhance the drama. From the viewpoint of the mental health practitioner whose patient has been caught up in this system, you need only know that a crime involves a violation of a criminal statute and the combination of a wrongful act (**actus reus**) and wrongful intent (**mens rea**). You may be called in at various stages of the proceedings to provide mitigating data based on mental illness, to aid in sentencing, to contribute to a probation program, to provide postrelease treatment at the end of a sentence, and so on; more formal questions (e.g., criminal responsibility) are ordinarily left to forensic specialists.

The civil system also involves clinicians, not only as potential **defendants** in a malpractice suit but also as other types of witnesses discussed in previous chapters in this volume. For clinicians, the most relevant aspect of civil litigation is **tort law,** which addresses wrongs done by one person to another and the mechanisms of compensation for the resultant injury. Note that if the injury claimed by a patient of yours is emotional or mental, your psychiatric evaluation and **testimony** may constitute an important part of the proceedings.

Torts are customarily divided into intentional torts (sins of commission) and unintentional torts (sins of omission). *Negligence* is a subset of the latter, where the claim is advanced that the defendant (target of the claim) neglected to do something such that he or she fell below the level of ordinary care—what the average person should have foreseen and taken action to prevent. For example, if there is ice on your sidewalk, it is foreseeable that someone may slip and fall, and thus ordinary care means doing something reasonable about it: ice removal, spreading sand, posting a warning sign, and so forth.

Professional negligence is a subset of the former category, whereby the clinician is compared not with the "average person" but with his or her peer group as a reference standard. Hence the conduct of the mental health professional—be it action or inaction—is compared with that of the average reasonable practitioner in that discipline, at the time and under the circumstances. Regional variations and embellishments of this standard abound.

Now we examine the steps along the sometimes years-long Via Dolorosa that lead to the **adjudication** malpractice suit. The idea was introduced earlier that a malpractice suit results from the malignant synergy of a bad outcome and bad feelings.[2] The mere fact that something bad happened does not in and of itself account for patients and clients choosing to become **plaintiffs** and file lawsuits. In fact, sad to say, these persons typically seek out an attorney only after their attempts to set things right with their treaters have been rebuffed.

Another important notion in the law is that of who bears the **burden of proof** in a given case and what the threshold of proof may be. In criminal cases—in which all persons are innocent until proven guilty—the "state," represented by a prosecutor, bears the burden of proving guilt **beyond a reasonable doubt.** Scholars sometimes depict this abstraction as a 95%–99% certainty that an individual is in fact guilty.

Similarly, the plaintiff bears the burden in civil cases, which are usually decided by a standard of **preponderance of the evidence,** probabilistically portrayed as "more likely than not," which is any level of certainty exceeding 50%—a far lower standard than in criminal cases. Certain other types of civil matters are decided by an intermediate standard of **clear and convincing evidence,** sometimes described as requiring approximately 75% certainty. Examples in some **jurisdictions** include termination of parental rights and involuntary **civil commitment.**

Before the Suit Is Filed

A few points should be made about your early and later responses that are sometimes overlooked. First, repairing the therapeutic alliance may well be possible at earlier stages of the game, such as when a patient protests that you have treated him or her badly, when your records are requested by a patient (or even when these are requested by an attorney—be sure to seek legal consultation on how to proceed in this particular instance), or when you hear indirectly that a patient is dissatisfied with your care.[2]

At those initial points of contact, discussion, conflict resolution, resumption of treatment, and, under some circumstances, careful apology may be not only indicated but also desirable. Bear in mind that a properly expressed apology immediately after a disaster has averted more suits than one can imagine.[3,4]

However, *after* the lawsuit has been filed, no matter how tempting it may be, *do not* attempt to reach or talk to your patient to find out the problem or even to dissuade him or her somehow from suing you; it is now too late for that. With the actual filing of the lawsuit, such forms of outreach are strictly contraindicated; the situation has become formal and adversarial, and legal counsel monitors and advises on everything prospectively. All contacts should flow through the attorneys from this point on.

Note carefully that at this and at almost every subsequent stage of the proceedings, an offer of settlement may be made. We have both even been retained in cases in which settlement was reached midtrial—before we even got to the stand. The essence of settlement is that the defendant pays a sum of money to the plaintiff, and the case goes away—that's all. Almost always, a settlement implies no admission of wrongdoing and thus seems like an excellent way to get on with your life. That, however, is the rub.

When we first entered the forensic field and observed malpractice litigation from the inside, our initial position in advising sued clinicians was typically to "fight this case to the highest court available; never give up." As experience grew, we became impressed with the emotional devastation and crushing blow to clinicians' morale that a malpractice suit can represent, even a baseless one. Our position shifted: in many cases we became advocates of settlement to get cases off the clinicians' backs so they could get on with their lives.

The newest change regarding litigation involving practitioners is the National Practitioner Data Bank. The obligatory reportage of every settlement, no matter how small, has somewhat shifted the balance of decision making. Some experts argue that it now pays to fight every case because if you win, nothing is reported, and if you lose, you are no worse off than you would be had you settled up front. Although it is true that winning a case keeps your slate clean with the data bank, we suggest that serious consideration still be given to settlement. It is unavoidably true that you will have to explain the suit to every future employer, but this may be worth it in the long run if the suit is predicated on an appropriately minor problem—for example, an unexpected allergic reaction to prescribed medication or a relatively inconsequential error in psychological test scoring.

First Contact

The first news you hear about litigation may be the dreaded letter from the lawyer, which may take several forms. In one version, the attorney simply states that a suit is being brought by Mr. Jones and requests that you notify your insurer. In another, the letter outlines every detail of the claim and the allegations supporting it. In any case, when this letter arrives, recall that the time for negotiating is past, and you must be guided strictly by your attorney to whom all communications from now on must be referred. Failure to follow this rule may jeopardize your case, handicap counsel's efforts on your behalf, and (Heaven forbid!) render your insurer free to pull out of funding your defense.

The Tribunal or Its Equivalent

To deal with the recent malpractice explosion, many jurisdictions have set up various forms of screening devices in a well-intentioned effort to screen out trivial or frivolous cases. In some areas, the attorney must obtain a report from a board-certified practitioner that the case has merit on the surface (i.e., assuming the claims are true and provable). Other areas use a tribunal, a quasi-judicial hearing in which the case is given a dry run. Tribunals may consist of attorneys and judges or may be a mixed membership of, for example, a physician, a lawyer, and a layperson.

Unfortunately, there is no guarantee that the mental health practitioner on some tribunals, for example, will practice in the same specialty area as the defendant. In practice, in our experience, tribunals actually serve to screen out only the most transparently baseless of claims (e.g., "That clinician's Trilafon caused me to lose my psychic powers"), but many frivolous ones get through nonetheless. Even if the tribunal makes a determination against the plaintiff, mechanisms often exist for going ahead with the case anyway, such as by posting a bond for court costs in advance and similar provisions.

Filing the Suit

The suit is filed in the form of a complaint against the defendant. At this juncture, the fact that you are being sued becomes a matter of public record. In responding, the defense team may engage in some combination of several potential maneuvers, typically denying some or all specific aspects of the complaint's contents and then making motions to dismiss the suit based on statute of limitations (the suit has been filed too late according to law), failure to state the claim for which relief can be granted (the allegations do not fit the mold of medical malpractice), and similar arguments.

Discovery Phase

The discovery phase is the point at which both sides research the case to determine what the facts are, what the strong and weak points of the case are, and what the potential experts on both sides think about it. The ultimate purpose of this process is to determine whether a settlement can be reached—either drop or settle—or whether proceeding to trial is the only possibility. In addition to simply obtaining relevant records, attorneys are permitted to pose certain questions in writing to the other side.

The answers to these **interrogatories**—which your lawyer will work closely with you to answer—are provided under **oath** and require as scrupulous accuracy of testimony as that in court. Depositions (also covered in considerable detail in Chapter 6, "'*Now* Do I Get My Say?'") are also part of the process. Various maneuvers and countermaneuvers may be initiated by attorneys to determine which questions will not be answered, which depositions will not be taken, and so on. If all settlement efforts fail, a trial will follow.

In almost every case, the attorneys retained by your insurer are top-notch and supportive as well as knowledgeable. We recommend avoiding the temptation, regardless of the stress you feel, to call your attorney every 4 days—or four times a day—to see how the case is progressing. Your attorney will call you when any developments worth noting occur. A lot of "hurry up and wait" is associated with litigation, so do not be surprised if months pass without a word.

The Trial Phase

If all settlement offers fail, the matter eventually goes to trial, the more detailed mechanics of which we examine later in this chapter. If you prevail at trial, the matter is resolved unless an **appeal** or claim of mistrial prolongs the ordeal. If the plaintiff wins, your insurer may try to negotiate payment of a sum of money—not necessarily what the jury awarded.

Aftermath

Either outcome—win or lose—at trial must be reported to the National Practitioner Data Bank. Practically, this means that you will be obliged to list and explain this event in future credentialing procedures. This task is burdensome but may not be problematic. In any case, you will do your best to get on with your life.

Specific Roles for the Clinician as Witness

The mental health professional will play a variety of roles in court beyond the general ones outlined earlier in this book. In this section, we focus on some special cases illustrating the difficulties associated with those roles that can be anticipated in court.

When Your Patient Sues You

The core situation in which this book is designed to be of help is when your patient sues you. Few experiences are as demoralizing as having your patient—in whom you have invested effort, time, skill, patience, and tolerance—turn around and sue you for alleged malpractice. Powerful and often unexpected feelings are stirred: outrage at the patient's apparent ingratitude, narcissistic injury, neurotic guilt, grief, depression, panic attacks, imagined shame in your colleagues' eyes, obsessive self-scrutiny to try to find out what you may have done wrong, and full-fledged hatred of the system. Practitioners who have not been sued find it hard to imagine the emotional devastation that can flow from even a baseless suit.

This emotional turmoil is triggered by the first formal notification that a suit has been brought against you. This notice may be called a demand letter, a claim letter, a legal complaint, or in some sites, a consumer complaint. The language of such letters, although usually standardized and dictated by custom, **regulation,** or statute, appears to depict you as having the medical competence of a flatworm, the social standing of pond scum, and the moral posture of an ax murderer. You are being put on notice that you are expected to drain your savings in atonement for the horrible things you are supposed to have done. At such moments, it may be all but impossible to recall that the language of these letters is, in a sense, as much a matter of rote theatricality as an attorney's posturing in the courtroom.

Note that patients or clients who sue their treaters sometimes appear to wish to continue treatment with them. This is a logical paradox but not a clinical one because litigation may serve several complex motivations, not all of which require cessation of treatment. However, the stresses, conflicts, legal pitfalls, and loss of objectivity that come with a malpractice suit preclude resuming or continuing treatment during pendency of the suit.[2]

When the time comes to testify as defendant with the patient present in the courtroom, a respectful demeanor and tactful modes of expression should be the rule, despite the emotions you may feel.

When Your Patient Sues Someone Else

In today's highly litigious society, it is not uncommon for your patient or client to be the plaintiff in litigation against another party. It could be a civil suit regarding a motor vehicle accident, a slip-and-fall case in a restaurant or grocery, divorce and child custody, or even a malpractice suit against another clinician.

If a patient or client claims to have endured emotional injuries, he or she may waive the applicable **privilege** so that a complete mental health history enters the process. Important implications of this development may include your discussing with the person whether opening up this door is truly advisable. Specific aspects of this role may include your reviewing psychotherapy notes to anticipate potentially embarrassing material and continuing your supportive role throughout litigation. You will resist any temptation to demonize the other side of the case or draw expert witness–type conclusions about the **damages** to the patient or client. Alteration of records in anticipation is strictly prohibited; such behavior would form the basis for a lawsuit in and of itself.

As noted earlier, a pitfall for many clinicians is to extend their representations beyond their own databases into the real world in which they were not actually present as witnesses. The entire body of information from the patient, in other words, can be described in terms of what the patient or client "says," "reports," "claims," "states," "maintains," "conveys," and so on. Although we generally believe what our patients tell us for therapeutic purposes, please recall that the courtroom requires a higher **standard of proof.**

This higher standard of proof becomes all the more critical in cases of posttraumatic stress disorder (PTSD), which is widely and appropriately regarded as a legal minefield.[5,6] One reason that this diagnosis causes so much more concern than any of the others in DSM-IV-TR[7] is that PTSD posits an actual event—the trauma—as the cause of the presenting symptoms. Presuming a real event and linking causation are elsewhere absent from the deliberately atheoretical DSM.

In summary, mental health professionals must beware of assuming that they know what occurred outside the office, given that almost all the information they receive is from their patients' and clients' usually uncorroborated reports. The clinicians who overidentify with their patients and clients and who "just know" their patients are reporting accurately actually do these persons a disservice by weakening the clinician's own credibility and thus utility as a witness. In objective fact, these treaters *do not* know because they were not there. Treaters who take the attitude that "if my patients said it, it must be true" will become, ironically, their patients' worst enemy in court.

As a fact witness—a role in which you may wind up serving if the patient does claim emotional harms—you are certainly free to describe the signs and symptoms you observed, the diagnoses you made, and the interventions you performed; these rest within your legitimate purview in the case.

The Patient as Defendant

Civil Matters

It is quite conceivable that someone may find a reason to sue your patient. In virtually every instance, your role will be a supportive one as you help the patient or client to deal clinically with the stress of litigation. It is probably essential that you avoid nontherapeutic entanglement in the case—yet another matter best left to the lawyers. You often will find that longer-term therapeutic goals will need to be suspended while you treat shorter-term symptomatic responses to the legal process. You may have to accept this moratorium on psychotherapeutic exploration because lawsuits are usually so highly preoccupying that other matters simply must wait. Discuss this fact candidly with your patient or client and decide jointly whether to continue in any more than supportive work until the matter is resolved.

Criminal Matters

If your patient is charged with a crime, the matter may grow slightly more complex. Lawyers may attempt to pervert your knowledge of your patient to aid the legal process, for example, by attempting to fit your patient to the profile of a certain type of offender. Your testimony in this context will be extremely problematic because it not only may harm your patient but also—because, in the interests of justice, the court may order you to testify—may render irrelevant your patient's permission to testify.

It is advisable to delegate the various litigation-oriented assessments and opinions about your patients or clients to a forensic expert who is removed from the treatment context. This approach is both more ethically sound and more likely to preserve the clinical advances achieved via the treatment relationship.

Other Medicolegal Issues

Child Custody Battles

Recognized as the most malignant of legal situations, the custody battle requires comprehensive assessment skills, knowledge of child psychology, and expertise in other forensically oriented details that fall outside usual clinical practice. The issue of custody battles is beyond the scope of this volume; fortunately, much useful literature exists on this topic.[8,9] Consultative experience confirms that custody battle issues should be left to the specialist.

Involuntary Civil Commitment

For the inpatient clinician, involuntary civil commitment is a fairly common occurrence and one for which some form of courtroom testimony is eventually required. As invariably dictated by statute, concrete data about dangerousness are particularly relevant, including past instances of violence and episodes on the unit of seclusion or restraint.

Involuntary Treatment

Mental health professionals give **evidence** to courts or quasi-judicial tribunals regarding the competence of patients or clients to consent to or to refuse (usually pharmacological) treatment. Although competence is a *legal* finding ultimately determined by a court (usually but not always a probate court), a *clinical* opinion is almost always solicited as to an individual's competence and requisite indications for the treatment in question. The clinician should keep in mind several important issues about involuntary treatment.

First, please note that patients enjoy what all citizens do: a legal presumption of competence. In other words, we are all considered competent unless affirmatively proven otherwise. Mere admission to a psychiatric hospital does not refute this presumption.

A common sign of incompetence is overt denial of a well-established and extensively recorded mental illness. A patient or client who speaks knowledgeably about medication but denies its potential relevance to his or her own condition may not be able to make reasonable and personal cost-benefit determinations about treatment. Observations from the entire treatment team may be particularly useful and can be presented by the treating psychiatrist, although some judges will insist on direct testimony from other clinical staff as well.

Some jurisdictions use a **substituted judgment** standard[2] for involuntary treatment of persons no longer capable of conveying consent—for example, those in a coma. This standard seeks to determine what the currently incapacitated patient or client would want were he or she competent. A history of having continued to take medication while presumably restored to a competent baseline may be highly relevant and easy for the court to incorporate: when competent, the patient or client *did* seek treatment.

More formal competence determinations, such as competence to make a will, are best left to the forensic mental health specialist.

The Six P's of Trial Preparation

Preparing for trial is a complex and often strenuous process, even if you are not the defendant-clinician in a malpractice case. This preparation can be organized around six principles: preparation, planning, practice, pretrial conference, pitfalls, and presentation (Table 9–1).

TABLE 9–1.   THE "SIX P's" OF TRIAL PREPARATION

Preparation

Planning

Practice

Pretrial conference

Pitfalls

Presentation

---

1. *Preparation:* This, of course, is the basic and overarching element. You should gather all the information and review it for rapid, clear memory access. Review the case, review the chart, review your notes, and get all of the available material up front and at your fingertips.
2. *Planning:* Recall that courtroom appearances involve both time and stress. Be sure to clear enough time; courts are notoriously unreliable as to scheduling, despite what you may have heard about accommodating physicians' schedules: court tends to be "hurry up and wait." Plan with counsel the timing of your arrival at the courthouse. Arrange for transportation and for adequate coverage of your practice so that you won't be worried or preoccupied. Take care of yourself by not undertaking new projects or seeing new patients; instead, arrange for rest and reflection time, enjoyable activities, and recreation. Resist the temptation just to take your courtroom appearance in stride without appropriate preparation.
3. *Practice:* Although there is much about a trial that you cannot predict, the facts of the case and your consequent direct testimony usually will be more predictable. Do not be shy about practicing your testimony in front of counsel, who should probably be encouraging you to do so. Rehearse several different ways of making your main points and select those that seem clearest to your rehearsal audience.
4. *Pretrial conference:* It is essential that you meet with counsel (in court, at counsel's office, or at your office) immediately before you go on the stand

each day. This will enable you to find out what new facts or issues have come to light and what the emotional tone is in the courtroom. Do not accept evasion of such meetings. Some attorneys are surprisingly casual about this, suggesting that "Well, we're going on at 9:00 A.M., so why not come by the courthouse around, oh, say, 8:50. We'll have a cup of coffee; we'll chat." Don't hesitate to reply: "I'm sorry, that's unacceptable. I can meet with you at 8:00 in the morning in the courtroom conference room, or 7:30 P.M. in your office the night before, and we'll review my testimony so I'll be better prepared for what we're getting into."

5. *Pitfalls:* Remaining alert to pitfalls at trial means knowing in advance not only the weaknesses or limits of your testimony but also the critical legal point or precise statutory language on which some issue in the case may turn. In anticipation of **cross-examination,** such pitfalls can be explored by determining the following with counsel's assistance: What will the opposing attorneys try to get me to say? Where are the hot spots, the weak spots, the ambiguities in the case? What are the historical or evidentiary pitfalls? What are the skeletons in my own closet that might be used to impeach me by innuendo (that unfounded prior complaint; that arrest for picketing the nuclear plant)? Although this strategy is really up to your lawyer, students of jury decision making recommend that any such pitfalls or weaknesses should be brought up directly; if they are likely to be brought out by the other side during cross-examination, you can minimize their potential effect by stealing the opposition's thunder.[10]

6. *Presentation:* It is not enough that you know what happened because it's your case, and you have reviewed it so intensely. You also must consider how you are going to present this largely technical material to a lay audience of nonclinicians. How are you going to make clear to them your clinical judgment, your reasoning, and most of all, your underlying concern for your patient or client as reflected in every aspect of your delivery of care?

The six P's are certainly relevant to your potential roles as observer, treater, or plaintiff, but they are particularly critical if you are the defendant. We review several specific issues relevant to your appearance in court in the following discussions.

Preparing Your Attorney

What should be your role in preparing your attorney for the upcoming litigation? We use the term *your attorney* in this section because he or she might be your insurer's attorney when you are being sued for malpractice, or he or she might be the attorney for whose side you are testifying (e.g., your patient's attorney if your patient, as plaintiff, is claiming some form of emotional harm). In any case, you will need to educate your attorney by explaining the clinical (i.e., mental health) issues of the case. These might include diagnosis, psychotherapy, psychopharmacology, indications for hospitalization, and so on.

For some top-flight attorneys, this task is barely an issue, simply because from trial experience they know more psychiatry than do many psychiatrists in the United States. Other attorneys are starting more nearly from scratch and may require extensive educating. Do not begrudge this time or attempt to delegate the task to the expert witnesses, if any, on the case; it is time well spent by you and you alone. A properly prepared attorney is your best ally in court.

Demystification is also quite helpful. Many laypersons, including attorneys who are not familiar with psychotherapy, for example, may view it as something of a voodoo science, full of arcane terminology and mystical activities. Demystification may be needed over and above simple education.

Next, you can educate your attorney as to the limits of the data. An attorney may not fully grasp that symptoms and history are fundamentally self-reports that for most lawyers are tantamount to hearsay—only rarely does the clinician have externally validated evidence for the facts that have been alleged. You may need to explain that a patient's or client's report is not proof. Moreover, there are limits to the amount of independent corroboration you can obtain without sacrificing the therapeutic alliance.

Finally, a challenging part of attorney preparation is your own awareness and alertness to various pressures and seductions that accompany going to court. You need to be alert to the fact that there will be time pressures to develop opinions before all the data are in, patient or client pressures to give favorable testimony, and seductions—monetary, narcissistic, and others— aimed at trying to convince you to do or say various other things. Mental health professionals who work closely with attorneys report how a growing identification with the attorney and with the attorney's position is a natural concomitant of the close working relationship. It is critical to keep this relational phenomenon from biasing your testimony. The issue transcends **perjury,** becoming an ethical mandate: the truth, the whole truth, and nothing but the truth, including the limits of data and areas of ignorance.

Dressing for Success

A surprisingly important issue is how you dress. Lecture audiences occasionally balk when we make this point, arguing that giving any weight to how you dress is unfair, unjust, petty, shallow, and ultimately irrelevant to your knowledge and professional skills. Some members of the audience will sputter, "But—a turtleneck sweater—that's who I am!" Our response is, perhaps so, but in the real world of the courtroom, in the glare of attention, you want every advantage you can obtain, every nuance in your favor—including how you appear.

To grasp this issue, consider what might be called "Chanel's Law," attributed to designer Coco Chanel in a movie. The quote (we cannot vouch for its accuracy or authenticity, but it captures the point perfectly) is: "Dress shabbily, they notice the dress; dress impeccably, they notice the woman." We add, "Dress unremarkably, they notice the testimony." To make the point clearer, anything that calls attention to your mode of dress or personal ornamentation is a distraction from what you have to say and therefore a bad idea. The implication is that the least-distracting mode of dress is conservative, although, for your comfort, it should be comfortably old and "broken in" (do *not* buy new suits for appearing in court).

Men and women should dress essentially like the lawyers they see in court and in the media. For men, a suit and tie are preferable because in some parts of the United States, a sports jacket, turtleneck, or the absence of a tie may connote an excessively casual attitude or even disrespect. Women should avoid dresses, pants, and shorts as well as high-heeled shoes and flats. Stick with the business suit and the medium-heel business shoe, and you won't go wrong.

Avoid ostentation. Leave the diamond-studded Rolex watch at home, and wear the rubber Timex in court; avoid elaborate dangling earrings, dramatic jewelry, multiple bracelets and chains, and electric colors. A wonderful literary example of the effect of dress on attention can be seen in the John Waters movie *Serial Mom* with Kathleen Turner. In one of the scenes in which she is defending herself at trial, Kathleen Turner is so distracted by the fact that one of the jurors has committed the fashion gaffe of wearing white shoes after Labor Day that she loses her entire train of thought.

In addition to dressing conservatively, you should turn off mobile phones and pagers when you enter the courtroom. Jurors are commonly annoyed at these interruptions during testimony (and may interpret them as arrogant demonstrations of how busy and important you think you are), but we have known judges to become enraged: the electronic intrusion is seen as disrespect of the court, which is perilously close to contempt. A word to the wise…

After you are suitably attired and sufficiently electronically neutralized, the next step is to take the witness stand. The most important principles are examined in the following sections.

Deposition Language Versus Trial Language

In your deposition, the court reporter was the most important party and constituted your audience because he or she was preparing your written record, the essence of the deposition. In keeping with this fact, your deposition answers were designed to be question-containing, short, austere yet complete, and well aimed at your audience of one. At trial, by contrast, your audience is the judge or jury. In this arena, *what* you say is almost less important than *how* you say it. For example, there may be occasions when a slightly *less* precisely accurate explanation for how something works may be preferable if it is more understandable to a lay jury audience.

In keeping with this change in audience, if you are asked a question at trial, answer that question until you have made your point to completion. Take as long as you need without filibustering or rambling. If someone grows impatient and rudely interrupts you, your credibility is unaffected because you are the person who has been interrupted while trying to give testimony, and everyone gets mad at—or more suspicious of—the attorney. If someone says, "Tell us how you understood the patient's problem," answer that question until you are completely through.

Of course, this approach has some practical limits (only so many days are allotted for a trial), and you certainly don't want to put the jury to sleep. Indeed, the slightest hint of jury squirming or the dreaded "eye-glaze" response is cause for bringing your discourse to a speedy resolution.

Another kiss of death during trial testimony occurs when you as the witness do not sound particularly interested in what you are saying. This situation can create an unspoken juror mentality such as "Look, you're actually involved in this case, and I'm just a juror; why should I be interested if you're not?"

Graphics and the Blackboard

As noted elsewhere in this book, the essential function of the clinician as witness is to teach; hence a tremendous benefit accrues from skillful use of graphics and the blackboard or flip chart. These devices have certainly been helpful in most lecture-style teaching, but the reason these methods are particularly effective in the courtroom is because of what might be called the *paracommunication effect.*

Laypersons, including jurors, may harbor all kinds of feelings about clinicians in general; such feelings are variations on the theme of transference, influenced by actual previous experience with internists, pediatricians, gynecologists, and mental health professionals. Although your demeanor on the witness stand will be the ultimate determinant of the jury's reaction to you, most juries have generally positive feelings about clinicians; however, some might have negative ones. Among these negative feelings, a common one is that clinicians do not talk to their patients enough or express enough of their decision making as it affects their patients' or clients' welfare.

In court, you will be doing exactly this: talking to the jury and explaining your reasoning. Properly handled, this explaining can be gratifying to jurors and can give them a break from the talking-heads monotony of the trial.

In addition, when you pick up a piece of chalk in your hand and stand in front of the blackboard, you become, as a transference object, the most trusted figure in common human experience: the teacher. The teacher *knows*. The juror may not know what the capital of Virginia is—or what chlorpromazine is used for—but knows that the teacher knows. The power of this image transcends what you actually draw; what counts is the apparent effort to get your point across because juries respond to the idea that you are *trying* to help them understand. Thus, whenever it may clarify a point, don't hesitate to use the blackboard or flip chart. Using these devices and what you will draw or list should be reviewed with your attorney in advance, of course, to permit the attorney's intelligent exploration of the issue.

Obviously, you should take pains to draw and write large enough for easy visibility and should resist the gaffe of talking to the blackboard instead of to the judge or jury as you speak.

Time to Testify

What about testimony itself? When asked a question, pause just a moment before answering. This brief delay permits you to replay the question in your head, ensure that you understand it, and allow your attorney to object if desired. That momentary pause is really important; you may not even have to answer the question if the objection is sustained. To keep the jury clear on what is happening, try to look thoughtful while you are thinking or even say—if you have to think about the answer a bit—"Well, I'd like to take just a moment to think about that." This statement keeps the jury from interpreting your silence as utter bafflement or as that you dozed off in midtrial—neither view redounding to your credit or credibility.

No one is usually bothered when you ask for time to think—you won't "look dumb" for having to do so—because it shows that you are taking your testimony seriously.

The Words You Say

The most vital tightrope you must walk during your trial testimony is the one stretched between being clear and being patronizing. Your use of basic, jargon-free English is absolutely essential, yet you must never talk down (or even seem to talk down) to the jury. One of our colleagues, testifying on *Court TV*, told a criminal trial jury that "my job was to disconfirm the hypothesis." This would stupefy almost any jury.

Why are your words so important? You might lose the jury for a moment or two, but you can eventually clear up any misunderstandings, can't you? In fact, the answer is no. There *is* an opportunity for redirect examination; however, the issue is not just a matter of dealing with the jury's lack of understanding. Going over the jury's head is alienating and antagonizing, and you may be given no chance to recover the jury's good opinion, regardless of whether you can correct a factual error.

How should you handle technical terms? Is there some way to explain *dysthymia* without using that term? How do you describe borderline personality disorder to a jury when some mental health professionals don't even understand it? Practice with a critical audience goes a long way to help you express these complex ideas in simple but not overtly or obviously simplistic ways.

If, despite your good intentions and conscientious rehearsal, you find yourself lapsing into jargon, define the term after you use it without making too big a deal of it. Explain terminology as part of your narrative, and don't make a production of doing so.

Wrong

WITNESS (pompously): After careful and meticulous observation, I made the diagnosis of dysthymia; now, you probably don't know what that means, and why should you? It is a term that we trained psychiatrists use to describe what the uninformed would term a depression lasting…

Better

WITNESS: I thought my patient was suffering from dysthymia, a long-lasting depression, and I…

Note that the description of dysthymia is a bit casual but not necessarily wrong; if it is important to fill in the details, that question will be asked later. The point here is that a bit of jargon that crept in was smoothly defined in an offhand, nonpatronizing manner.

During the previously mentioned "momentary pause," it is a given that you will think before you speak. As a concomitant of this idea, don't shoot from the hip and don't trip on your own ego, especially in thinking that you know it all. A common example of shooting from the hip is when you really don't know the answer but are willing to guess or to speculate by extrapolation from your usual procedure, for example. Resist this temptation. This practice is extremely dangerous. It is far better to say, "I don't know" or "I don't recall," even if you fear that will make you sound foolish. That is a far sounder position to be in than having to retract that guess or speculation on cross-examination when the inquiring attorney is not your ally.

In court you are, of course, aware of the plaintiff and the defendant and who is who, but recall that those terms are depersonalized. As a rule, you should *not* refer to the parties by those names. You want to express yourself in vivid, functional terms: "My patient, Ms. Jones" (not "the plaintiff"); "I consulted Dr. Johnson" (not "my codefendant"). Some witnesses can get away with referring to "poor Ms. Jones" to convey their sympathy: she is a suffering person, not just a pawn in the legal game. Be careful with any attempts to use this brand of locution because it could sound sarcastic or patronizing—especially if the patient or client is on the other side of the case from you. Never, however, use patients' first names; this will sound either demeaning or excessively intimate, neither of which aids your presentation. Use last names and honorifics even if, in reality, you were always on a first-name basis with the patient.

Pitfalls and Hot Spots

Although experience is inevitably the best teacher of how to handle trial testimony, there are some points that might stave off the more egregious difficulties.

Witness Fees

As is the case in psychotherapy and billing practices, money can be a sensitive issue on the witness stand. Fact witnesses are usually paid no fee for their time or a token "**subpoena** fee" (e.g., in Massachusetts, this is a generous $8.00 one-time honorarium). Their participation as witnesses in the judicial system is considered a part of their civic responsibility, like jury duty. If you are the treating clinician testifying on behalf of your patient or client, you are free to negotiate a fair rate with your patient; occasionally, an attorney will agree to pay you an expert hourly fee, despite your fact witness role, even though the rationale for doing so is pretty flimsy. If this arrangement will govern, get something in writing about it before trial. Because of the clinical and ethical conflicts involved, you should not attempt to solve this problem by functioning as an expert if you are already the treater. Whatever arrangement is made, acknowledge it frankly on the stand if asked.

Never and Always

Predictably, the terms *never* and *always* are land mines disguised as ordinary words. They also could be described as empty sets because few things in psychiatry or psychology, at least, are never or always true. You will not go wrong if you regard any question containing these terms as a trap. Use them sparingly if at all in your own testimony.

Misquotation of Your Testimony

Inaccurate or slightly distorted quotes of your previous testimony are a common ploy. For example, if the opposing attorney says, "Doctor, do you remember before when you testified that physicians were free to abuse every patient they see?," you might say, "I have to admit, counselor, although that doesn't sound familiar to me, I do recall commenting on how difficult it was for physicians to police themselves." Just because the attorney begins a query with your previous testimony does not mean that what comes out is really what you said; the lawyer is not under oath. Assuming automatically that the lawyer is quoting you accurately is dangerous.

Subordinate Clauses as a Foot in the Door

Let us examine another technical point that may be useful in giving complete testimony. Assume for the moment that your answer, in the previous example, omitted the "although." Thus, "I have to admit, counselor, that doesn't sound familiar to me." You then draw in your breath to continue with "I do recall…," but at this point, the attorney would be within his or her rights to interrupt you and say, "That's all right if you don't remember what you said, Doctor, you've answered the question, and the record will speak for itself." Note how this latter version makes you seem to have a poor memory at best or to wish to retract sworn testimony at worst. By beginning your answers with the all-important subordinate clause ("Although that doesn't sound familiar to me, I do recall…"), you effectively compel the questioner to wait for the end of the completed answer, lest he or she seem to be interrupting you.

Simple Harassment

A classic saying attributed to Cicero exhorts lawyers to this effect: "When the facts are in your favor, argue the facts; when the facts are not in your favor, yell and pound on the table." Our own experience suggests that as a witness you have less to fear from the screaming table pounders than from the soft-spoken, scrupulously polite advocates who lead you down the garden path without your realizing it.

Fortunately for you as a witness, lawyerly harassment tends to occur far less often than television and movies would suggest. Lawyers are actually concerned with seeming to be too harsh toward the witness, and judges are usually pretty sensitive as well to the occasional need for "protection" of the fact witness. In fact, despite the ever-popular courtroom drama cliché wherein the attorney is screaming abusive questions into the cowering witness's face from a range of 6 inches, most of the time lawyers are not even allowed to approach you on the witness stand without both good cause and the judge's permission.

Nonetheless, you should be prepared for harassment, with the explicit goal of not letting it touch you at all. Let it bounce off, the way that you might if a patient or client were screaming at you that you are an incompetent therapist. It has nothing to do with you or your testimony. Moreover, maintaining your cool has a positive effect on your presentation before the jury. Conversely, of course, losing your cool has the opposite effect.

Impugning Your Pretrial Preparation

Attorneys may attack you for your engaging in preparation prior to trial: "Doctor, isn't it true that you met with your attorney just before appearing on this stand?" The idea behind this query is that you are somehow being coached and that your testimony is inauthentic. The truthful response is always best. You might respond, "Of course, I did; I insist on meeting with my attorney because that's what my lawyer is for—to help me understand these proceedings."

Nonblissful Ignorance

Most psychiatrists cherish a deep resistance to admitting on the witness stand that they do not understand a question or do not know an answer; like most other resistances, this one must be overcome. Do not be afraid to say, "I don't understand the question" or "I don't know the answer to that." It is the lawyer's job to ask you a question in a form or a manner that you can understand; if you don't, the attorney should rephrase the question or ask something else. Similarly, no one remembers everything. If an attorney needs you to recall something for subsequent queries, he or she may show a document.

If you don't recall a fact needed to answer a question, but you know where to look it up in the medical records in front of you on the witness stand, it is appropriate to offer, "I don't recall that, but I think I can find it in just a moment." If it is critical, most attorneys will let you look it up. They also may show you a blowup of the chart or make a "representation" about the point. This means that the attorney is supplying the missing fact in order to move on to the next question; for example: "Doctor, let me represent to you that the August 1st discharge summary gives a final diagnosis of schizophrenia. Would it surprise you then to learn…?"

Remember that if you really do not recall, do not guess or infer. If the point is truly important, the lawyer can find it and show it to you so that you can give an informed and valid answer.

The Presence of the Patient or Client

Even when your patient or client is the litigant, he or she may not be present at all times in the courtroom. Either way, respectful language should be maintained with utmost of care. You would never say: "I diagnosed Mr. Jones as a typical common thug of the born-loser variety." You would say, instead, "Mr. Jones described a lengthy history of antisocial acts and incarcerations." The approach of objectivity is best achieved by stating the facts plainly and simply.

Even for the trial-seasoned witness, going to court is rarely an unalloyed pleasure. Some familiarity with the overt and latent issues and some introduction to the foundational techniques discussed in this chapter may at least mitigate the more traumatic aspects.

• **Key Points**

- • Trials are the culmination of what may be literally years of alternately plodding and hurried events; we need to track and come to understand these events as closely as possible to derive the most appropriately favorable outcomes.

- • Our own courtroom appearances are best served by an optimal approach to preparation, planning, practice, pretrial conferencing, anticipating pitfalls, and presenting ourselves in the most adaptive fashion.

- • Personal details such as dress, style of speech, and overall comportment become highly significant in the sensitive and high-stakes atmosphere of the courtroom, with the proceedings almost always preserved as a permanent and potentially revisited audio or video record.

References

1. Garoupa N: The syndrome of the efficiency of the common law. Boston University International Law Journal 29:287–335, 2011
2. Appelbaum PS, Gutheil TG: Clinical Handbook of Psychiatry and the Law, 4th Edition. Baltimore, MD, Lippincott, Williams & Wilkins, 2007
3. Gutheil TG: On apologizing to patients. Risk Management Foundation Forum 8:3–4, 1987 (Contact the Risk Management Foundation at 617-495-5100.)
4. Fehr R, Gelfand MJ: When apologies work: how matching apology components to victims' self-construals facilitates forgiveness. Organ Behav Hum Decis Process 113:37–50, 2010
5. Simon RI (ed): Posttraumatic Stress Disorder in Litigation: Guidelines for Forensic Assessment, 2nd Edition. Washington, DC, American Psychiatric Publishing, 2003
6. Stone AA: Post-traumatic stress disorder and the law: critical review of the new frontier. Bull Am Acad Psychiatry Law 21:23–36, 1993
7. American Psychiatric Association: Diagnostic and Statistical Manual of Mental Disorders, 4th Edition, Text Revision. Washington, DC, American Psychiatric Association, 2000

8.   Cooke G, Norris DM: Child custody and parental fitness, in Handbook of Forensic Assessment: Psychological and Psychiatric Perspectives. Edited by Drogin EY, Dattilio FM, Sadoff RL, et al. Hoboken, NJ, Wiley, 2011, pp 433–458

9.   Galatzer-Levy R, Krauss L, Galatzer-Levy J (eds): The Scientific Basis of Child Custody Decisions. Hoboken, NJ, Wiley, 2009

10. Williams KD, Bourgeois MJ, Croyle RT: The effects of stealing thunder in criminal and civil trials. Law Human Behav 17:597–609, 1993

CHAPTER 10

"Do I Still Get to Have a Life?"

Self-Care During Litigation

BEING SUED casts a long shadow over one's life, seeming at times to dominate every waking thought. Despite facile reassurances from well-meaning friends and colleagues that "this happens to everyone," "the insurer will handle it," "the suit is probably bogus," and so on, you will not be in the most sanguine of moods during the course of litigation.

Dealing with this kind of stress requires attention to several factors to prevent the process from wreaking havoc with work, family, and physical and mental health. Although there is no way to turn this experience into fun, we offer some time-tested approaches to surviving the storm, continuing to practice your profession, preserving your sanity, and maintaining a good relationship with your family and friends. The core principle is to preserve those aspects of life that promote well-being while allowing for the inevitable disruptions that litigation will produce.

Time Management

Two common extremes we see in our consultative practice might be labeled as "hurry up" and "stop." The first involves throwing oneself into a frenzy of activity to take one's mind off the threat; the second involves bringing one's entire life to a dead halt. As you have already guessed, neither approach is adaptive.

Clinicians who are being sued appear to lose the thread of appropriate time management in several observable ways. First, we need to recognize that time itself is a finite resource. The mechanics and logistics of being sued inescapably require a substantial allotment of this precious commodity. It takes time to review your entire history of care, to immerse yourself in the record, and to catch up on as much of the relevant literature as possible. Meeting with your insurer's attorney—or your own, for that matter—also takes time, and this obligation cannot be scanted in favor of procrastination.[1]

One valuable principle will help considerably: *no new burdens*. Rather than filling time, your goal should be clearing time. That means not taking on many new patients or assuming new responsibilities. Try to delay that promotion to a more demanding position. Put off plans to write that article on a nonessential topic that always intrigued you. Postpone that cross-country lecture tour.

Preserve the Basics

The three activities most likely to be affected and disrupted by the stress of litigation are paradoxically the most essential to preserving and promoting your viability as a legal client, litigant, and functional witness: eating, sleeping, and exercise. Conscious efforts should be devoted to maintaining a healthy diet, allowing sufficient sleep time, and continuing—or starting—an exercise regimen.[2] Actively resist the temptation to let these activities slide because of your preoccupation with the lawsuit ("I'll tough it out").

Vacations, Hobbies, and Leisure Activities

Most **defendants** insist that they cannot even think of indulging themselves in vacations, hobbies, or leisure activities because they must remain poised to respond to the demands of litigation. Although fully understandable, this is an unrealistic view. Any attainable moments of relaxation are worth their weight in gold.

Here again, conscious efforts should be made to follow familiar routines. Travel to favorite local spots. Attend movies, concerts, or plays. Maintain spiritual activities. Take family outings, ski trips, or picnics. Arrange for thoughtful coverage of your caseload, so you will not have to stay in constant touch with the office. It is always a good idea to tell your attorney if you will be out of touch for some time and to provide him or her with your contact data—for legal emergencies only.

Family and Friends

Our greatest support during times of adversity comes from family and friends. These relationships should be sustained, albeit with one important caveat. Spouses, for example, cannot typically be compelled to testify against you in criminal or civil cases, but most other individuals with whom you discuss your case could conceivably be dragged into court to testify about this—not exactly a situation designed to endear you to your inner circle. Always remember to practice some circumspection in your communications with others. A good rule of thumb here is "Feelings, yes; facts, no."

Use of social media represents another pitfall. The temptation to go to cyberspace with your story, especially if you think that the suit is especially false and frivolous, can be very strong, but resist that temptation too—even if you think you have somehow cleverly disguised the facts or parties involved.

Professional colleagues can be highly supportive in this situation because empathy and identification usually run high, but here again, maintaining the focus on your feelings rather than on trying to argue the case is the best approach. When asked under **oath** whether you discussed the case with colleagues, you can truthfully say that you discussed only how you personally felt about being the subject of litigation and not about its substance.

Safe Places to Discuss the Case

Defendant clinicians unable to vent their feelings about the case and the suit may feel like they are ready to explode, but fortunately, two main sources of support are available that are highly unlikely to be brought into court against you. The first is personal mental health treatment. Some clinicians nationwide have practices focused on helping sued clinicians cope with the strain. The value of such interventions cannot be overestimated; the content of such sessions is typically protected. The second is consultation with clergy.

Consult with counsel before availing yourself of these resources to ensure that you learn just how relevant protections may be functioning in your particular **jurisdiction** and with your particular type of case.

How Should I Manage My Practice?

A lawsuit casts its shadow over your clinical practice and your life in general. A mental health practitioner sued in connection with a patient's or client's suicide, for example, simply cannot escape being somewhat gun-shy when treating the depressed persons who surface in any typical caseload. The impulse toward overreaction is entirely understandable yet problematic. Moreover, your faith in your clinical judgment has been shaken to some extent by the fact of suit, no matter how baseless the accusations against you may be.

The challenge will be to attempt to continue practicing as carefully as always without massively altering your clinical approach. Here, recall that the mere fact of being sued does not mean you did something wrong. Reasonable risks cannot be avoided in the service of fostering patient responsibility and autonomy.

A useful approach to coping with the strain is active consultation or supervision.[3] You can pursue a narrow focus restricted to the most challenging patients or clients alone, or, alternatively, you can broaden this assistance to your entire caseload. Consultation or supervision not only provides some comfort and reassurance but also may serve as a check on simple errors made as a function of stress.

• **Key Points**

- Few of us will have the luxury of suspending our clinical activities in anticipation of a courtroom appearance, so we must continue practicing as carefully as always without massively altering our clinical approach.

- Basic self-care activities such as proper diet, sleeping, and exercise must continue throughout those stressful periods before and between direct encounters with the legal system.

- We should avoid becoming socially isolated while dealing with legal proceedings, but at the same time, we must remain cautious not to engage family and friends in discoverable discussions of the facts and allegations in question.

References

1. Gafni R, Geri N: Time management: procrastination tendency in individual and collaborative tasks. Interdisciplinary Journal of Information, Knowledge, and Management 5:115–125, 2010
2. Esch T, Stefano GB: The neurobiology of stress management. Neuro Endocrinol Lett 31:19–39, 2010
3. Wallbank S, Hatton S: Reducing burnout and stress: the effectiveness of clinical supervision. Community Pract 84(7):31–35, 2011

CHAPTER 11

"Where Do I Go From Here?"

The Aftermath of Litigation

NOW THAT the hurly-burly is done and your case is lost or won, you can take a deep breath and consider what you may have learned from all of this.

We hope you have realized that it is possible to learn even from a very adverse and possibly traumatic experience and that just because you have been sued does not mean that you are a bad doctor—although you may have found yourself feeling as if you were. You might even qualify for a diagnosis of posttraumatic stress disorder. If so, get into treatment, either as an individual or in a group with other sued clinicians. Professional organizations in many areas across the United States sponsor such groups, which can help counter the sense of isolation that comes with being singled out by the legal system.

You also may have learned a lot about anxiety. Anxiety, some say, is like blood pressure: everyone needs to have some, but too much and too little are both problematic. Too much anxiety interferes with good functioning, but an optimal level—not too much, not too little—may actually help you to learn, focus, and function better. In other words, you can take advantage of what you have been through. It may actually make you a better practitioner: more humane and effective, more attentive to your patients' emotional connection with you, and more attuned to the production of careful, efficient documentation. One of our main goals in writing this book has been to show practitioners how to make their understandable anxiety about litigation more manageable.

From here, your course is to return to the human being you were before fate called your number. This will involve picking up the parts of your life that you had to lay aside to deal with court: going back to getting more than 4 hours sleep a night, catching up with what your favorite sports team is doing these days, and reconnecting with your family.

You also will be dealing with some fairly predictable pitfalls along the way. How do you avoid overreacting when a new patient or client presents with the same clinical picture, the same illness or symptoms, as the patient who sued you? How do you keep from being gun-shy, excessively risk averse, and defensive and from overcompensating in ways that do not necessarily help your patient? It is probably wise to step up your level of consultation and supervision requests, at least in the short term, until you feel that you are back to your baseline. Don't forget to return to your regular exercise regimen and vacation schedules.

Life truly begins anew when the last **deposition** has been taken, the last hearing has been conducted, and the last order has been issued. No more outraged stares in dingy courtrooms from people you were only trying to help in the first place. No more semi-informed accusations in ornate boardrooms from people who still haven't grasped what your help really means. *You'll get there*—and we hope this book will help make your passage as predictable and tolerable as possible.

APPENDIX I

The Civil Litigation Process

Prefiling Settlement Negotiation

+ May also continue throughout the proceedings.

Filing and Service of the Complaint

+ Outlines the strongest case that the plaintiff can put forward on the basis of prediscovery evidence; "service" refers to the act of conveying the complaint to the relevant parties.

Response to the Complaint

+ Defendant addresses each element of the complaint.
+ Defendant may file a motion—typically, a written plea delivered to the court—to dismiss.

Note. Variations will occur on a regional or case-by-case basis. Special thanks to W. Foote, Ph.D., A.B.P.P., for his contributions to an earlier version of this outline.

Discovery

- Requests are made for document production, such as medical records.
- Subpoenas are issued for document production.
- Clinicians complete physical and/or mental examinations of plaintiffs or—at times—defendants.
- Interrogatories are answered.
- Depositions are scheduled.

Motions for Summary Judgment

- These motions are granted to parties who successfully prove that no genuine factual dispute exists on any legally salient issues, so there is no need to squander the court's resources by putting the case before a jury; for example, when the plaintiff transparently lacks a case, as in claiming that treatment has resulted in a "loss of psychic powers and extrasensory perception."

Pretrial Conference

- Witness and exhibit lists are exchanged.
- Discovery cutoff occurs, such that no new evidence can be requested from opposing parties.
- Additional pretrial motions are filed.

Ongoing Motion Practice

- Motions *in limine* request that potentially prejudicial information not be allowed to be heard in the interest of fairness.
- Motions for protective orders request that the court protect someone from further abusive service of process or discovery, such as personal inquiries designed to embarrass rather than to produce truly relevant evidence.

Trial Sequence

- Plaintiff presents "case in chief," laying out his or her case formally.
- Plaintiff attempts to meet burden of proof.
- Plaintiff rests.
- Defendant may move for a "directed verdict," by which device he or she wins the case automatically when the judge proclaims that the plaintiff's

case, as a matter of law, is insufficient to prevail; failure to obtain a directed verdict means the trial continues.

- Defendant presents "case in chief," laying out his or her case formally.

Posttrial

- Jury begins deliberations and determines verdict.
- Motion for judgment *non obstante veredicto* ("notwithstanding the verdict") may be ordered, by which device the judge can proclaim that one side or the other has actually won, as a matter of law, despite the jury having found otherwise—for example, the jury may have sided with one allegedly more sympathetic party in open defiance of the jury instructions.
- "Entry of judgment" formally establishes the trial's outcome.
- Motions for reconsideration are filed, in which the trial court is asked to alter its decision.
- The appellate process begins, in which a higher court is asked to modify the decision reached by the trial court.
- Settlement negotiations are renewed—although the trial is over, the parties still may have an opportunity, for example, to arrange that lesser compensation will be paid on an accelerated schedule.

| Prefiling settlement negotiation | → If successful, no suit will occur. |

↓

| Filing and service of the complaint |

↓

| Response to the complaint |

↓

| Discovery |

↓

| Motions for summary judgment | → If defendant's motions are successful, then the suit is dismissed. |

↓

| Pretrial conference | → If renewed negotiations are successful, then the trial may be averted. |

↓

| Ongoing motion practice | → If defendant's motions are granted, then some evidence may be excluded |

↓

| Trial sequence | → If defendant's motions are granted, then the trial may be terminated in defendant's favor; defendant also may simply win outright. |

↓

| Posttrial | → If outcome is unfavorable to defendant, then the decision may be appealed; reduced liability still may be negotiated. |

APPENDIX II

Legal Glossary

Actus reus   The specific physical act that a defendant must have committed to be found guilty of a crime (see *mens rea*)

Adjudication   The court's final determination in a legal disputed matter

Admissibility   The extent to which a court will permit a particular item into evidence for consideration by a judge or jury (see *relevance*)

Affirmation   An appellate court's conclusion that a lower court's decision is allowed to stand

Agency   The status of being authorized to act—or being considered as authorized to act—for another entity; for example, this may serve to extend criminal or civil liability to a hospital for your allegedly improper actions as its employee

Appeal   An attempt by a party subjected to a losing criminal or civil adjudication to have that decision overturned by a higher court

---

Source.   Adapted from Drogin EY, Dattilio FM, Sadoff RL, et al. (eds): *Handbook of Forensic Assessment: Psychological and Psychiatric Perspectives.* Hoboken, NJ, Wiley, 2011.

Appellate court   A higher court responsible for reviewing the decisions of a trial court or lower appellate court (see *affirmation*)

Attorney-client privilege   The protected status of communications between a lawyer and the persons he or she represents; disclosure of these communications cannot be compelled because of the legal system's recognition of the importance of a client's ability to consult confidentially with counsel (see *privilege*)

Beyond a reasonable doubt   Proven to an extent that seemingly affords little if any possibility of error; required for conviction in criminal matters (see *clear and convincing evidence, preponderance of the evidence*, and *standard of proof*)

Burden of proof   The responsibility for establishing that sufficient evidence exists for a criminal conviction or a finding of civil liability; this burden is typically ascribed to criminal prosecutors and civil plaintiffs (see *standard of proof*)

Case law   Presumptively binding legal principles that are established on the basis of prior appellate court decisions (see *precedent*)

Civil commitment   The process of compelling an individual to undergo inpatient or outpatient mental health treatment, in light of factors such as dangerousness to self or others, amenability to treatment, the likely efficacy of treatment, and the likelihood that the proposed setting for treatment is the least intrusive or confining option available

Clear and convincing evidence   Proven to an extent that appears unambiguous and reasonably compelling (see *beyond a reasonable doubt, preponderance of the evidence*, and *standard of proof*)

Common law   Precedents that are established by judicial decisions in the form of case law rather than by legislatively codified rules (see *statutory law*)

Confidentiality   The general expectation that a party receiving information will not disclose that information, its source, or the circumstances under which it was obtained (see *privilege*)

Conflict of interest   The presence of competing or otherwise incompatible obligations or opportunities; typically invoked to limit the questionably appropriate provision of professional services

Continuance   A delay of legal proceedings due to a formally asserted hardship or impracticality

Cross-examination   Counsel's initial elicitation of evidence through testimony, during deposition or trial, from the opposing side's witness in a criminal or civil case (see *direct examination*)

Damages   The nature of the harm occasioned by a civil defendant's allegedly inappropriate personal or professional conduct; this term is also used to refer to the financial penalties imposed on the basis of such harm (see *tort law*)

Defendant   A person legally accused of having violated criminal law or of having failed to meet civil standards for personal or professional conduct

Deposition   The documentation of evidence taken from a witness, usually by opposing counsel, prior to the occurrence of an actual criminal or civil trial; this is often conducted to obtain a sense of the potency of the evidence and the likely persuasiveness of the witness himself or herself

Direct examination   Counsel's initial elicitation of evidence through testimony, during deposition or trial, from his or her own witness in a criminal or civil case (see *cross-examination*)

Disposition   The ultimate outcome of criminal or civil proceedings (see *adjudication*)

Docket   A list of legal matters currently before an appellate or a trial court for its consideration

Evidence   Information from several sources offered in support of legal arguments in a criminal or civil matter

Expert witness   An individual whose knowledge, skill, education, training, and experience are considered sufficient for providing special assistance to the trier of fact, such that he or she is allowed to offer opinions on various issues before the court (see *fact witness*)

Fact finder   The role of a judge or jury in determining whether a factual allegation has actually been proven (see *burden of proof*)

Fact witness   An individual who observed the event in question or who otherwise has concrete information to share with the court; he or she is not answering hypothetical questions or otherwise opining in the role of an "expert"(see *expert witness*)

Felony   A serious criminal offense, typically punishable by imprisonment for 1 or more years or the imposition of a substantial fine (see *misdemeanor*)

Fine   A financial penalty levied by the court as a result of civil or criminal proceedings

Guardian ad litem   An attorney (or sometimes a clinician or even a layperson) who completes a wide range of functions intended to aid the court in gathering information

Impairment   A state of diminished mental capacity; this may result in a lack or diminution of criminal responsibility or civil liability

Informed consent   Granting permission for being subjected to a medical or psychological procedure after having been provided with sufficient knowledge about that procedure, delivered in suitably accessible language, with an opportunity to obtain answers to one's additional questions

Interrogatories   A series of highly specific questions, posed in writing to a witness in the early stages of a civil matter; counsel may ultimately advise the witness to refrain from answering some of these questions if they are irrelevant or otherwise exceed the scope of proper inquiry

Jurisdiction   The geographic area within which—or the subject matter concerning which—a particular court is deemed qualified to conduct criminal or civil proceedings

Liability   Exposure to the consequences of having violated either criminal law or civil standards for personal or professional conduct

Licensure   Formal recognition of the right to practice one's profession in a given jurisdiction, typically following some combination of written examination, oral examination, and certification that one is suitably licensed in another jurisdiction that adheres to similar standards for enabling professional practice

Locality rule   The process of setting the standard for appropriate professional practice at the level typically observed in one's own geographic area (see *malpractice, national standard,* and *negligence*)

Malpractice   The failure to provide services at a requisite level of professional competency; recall the "four D's" as found in the time-honored mnemonic, "Dereliction of a Duty Directly causing Damages" (see *locality rule, national standard,* and *negligence*)

Mens rea   The specific mental state that a defendant must have been experiencing in order to be found guilty of a crime (see *actus reus*)

Misdemeanor   A criminal offense typically punishable by imprisonment for less than 1 year or the imposition of a fine (see *felony*)

National standard   The process of gauging the appropriateness of one's practices at the level typically observed in the countrywide professional community (see *locality rule, malpractice,* and *negligence*)

Negligence   A criminally or civilly inappropriate failure to act as would a reasonable person in a given situation (see *malpractice*)

Oath   A formal statement of the truthfulness of one's assertions (see *perjury*)

Perjury   The proffer of deliberately untruthful information in the context of criminal proceedings (see *oath*); such activity is typically subject to criminal sanctions

Plaintiff   A party to a civil proceeding seeking redress for alleged harm (see *defendant*)

Precedent   The legal notion that prior appellate court decisions constitute binding guidance for future rulings on the same issues

Preponderance of the evidence   Proven to an extent that is even slightly more convincing than the arguments offered to the contrary (see *beyond a reasonable doubt, clear and convincing evidence,* and *standard of proof*)

Privilege   The right to bar from admission into legal or quasi-legal proceedings certain information or the circumstances under which such information was obtained; this is typically acknowledged—with various exceptions—in communications between attorneys and clients, between physicians and patients, and between spouses (see *confidentiality*)

Pro se   Undertaking to represent oneself or otherwise to seek a particular result from the court without representation by legal counsel

Proximate cause   Sufficient contribution to harm as to incur civil liability (see *tort law*)

Reasonable degree of certainty   That level of confidence in one's own opinion deemed necessary by various courts for the proffer of expert witness testimony

Rebuttal   The process of proffering evidence for the specific purpose of countering the assertions of a legal opponent's witnesses

Regulation   A legal rule promulgated by an administrative agency, typically in support of codified laws enacted by a legislative body (see *statute*)

Release   A signed document authorizing the proffer of sensitive information (see *confidentiality* and *privilege*)

Relevance   Sufficient utility for the tasks of a judge or jury for facts or assertions to be considered formally in the context of legal proceedings (see *admissibility* and *evidence*)

Respondent   An individual who has become the subject of civil proceedings—for example, when someone is the focus of a complaint to the state board of licensure

Restitution   Moneys ordered payable by a civil or criminal court to compensate the victim of a physical, emotional, or other injury (see *damages*)

Standard of care   The inferred quality of patient or client services typically expected in the pursuit of a particular profession (see *malpractice* and *standard of practice*)

Standard of practice   The inferred level of competency typically expected in the pursuit of a particular profession (see *malpractice*)

Standard of proof   The degree to which a party must establish the existence of certain facts or circumstances in order to prevail in a legal proceeding (see *beyond a reasonable doubt, clear and convincing evidence,* and *preponderance of the evidence*)

Statute   Codified legal guidance, instituted by a state or federal legislative body, the violation of which may result in criminal proceedings (see *regulation*)

Statutory law   Precedents that are established by legislatively codified rules rather than by judicial decisions in the form of case law (see *common law*)

Subpoena   A legal document directing that a witness appear in court, perhaps to produce a specified item of evidence; a subpoena may be overridden or "quashed" at the court's discretion if the document in question is premature, overreaching, or otherwise inappropriate

Substituted judgment   The legal process whereby a court will assume or delegate decision making for an individual because of that individual's relevant physical or mental incapacity and—under certain circumstances—previously expressed wishes

Testimony The rendering—typically sworn—of a witness's statements during a trial or deposition

Third party An entity—other than that suing or being sued—with some relevant relation to the legal matter at issue; for example, an insurer who may be financially liable for a civil defendant's improper actions

Tort law That body of legal guidance establishing a party's obligations to other persons under certain circumstances, with noncriminal penalties for inadequate compliance that often include providing financial compensation to injured parties; liability typically relies on the presence of a duty, a breach of that duty, harm to a victim as a result of that breach, and sufficient contribution to that harm (see *damages* and *proximate cause*)

Trial The forum in which opposing legal perspectives are formally aired, resulting in the rendering of a decision by a judge or jury

Trier of fact The role of the judge or jury in determining whether certain events or situations occurred or existed at a given time; this is distinct from determining whether an applicable legal standard has been met

Trier of law The role of the trial judge in determining whether an applicable legal standard has been met

Ultimate issue The actual legal matter that a court is attempting to determine; some jurisdictions maintain that expert witnesses should be prevented from addressing such matters directly—for example, that they should be allowed to opine on the presence or absence of relevant mental conditions and abilities but not on the presence or absence of competency or capacity

Verdict A legal determination that an accused party either has or has not committed a criminal act or has had a civilly actionable lapse in personal or professional conduct

Violation A breach of statutory, regulatory, or case law that may render an individual subject to criminal prosecution

Writ A court order directing or enabling a party to act in a prescribed fashion

APPENDIX III

Recommended Readings and Online Support

American Congress of Obstetricians and Gynecologists: Litigation Stress Resources. Available at: http://www.acog.org/About_ACOG/ACOG_Districts/District_IX/Litigation_Stress_Resources.

Barsky AE, Gould JW: Clinicians in Court: A Guide to Subpoenas. New York, Guilford, 2004

Bernstein BE, Hartsell TL: The Portable Lawyer for Mental Health Professionals, 2nd Edition. Hoboken, NJ, Wiley, 2004

Bernstein BE, Hartsell TL: The Portable Guide to Testifying in Court for Mental Health Professionals. Hoboken, NJ, Wiley, 2005

Brenner IR: How to Survive a Medical Malpractice Lawsuit: The Physician's Road Map for Success. Hoboken, NJ, Wiley, 2010

Charles SC, Frisch PR: Adverse Events, Stress, and Litigation: A Physician's Guide. New York, Oxford University Press, 2005

Choctaw WT: Avoiding Medical Malpractice: A Physician's Guide to the Law. New York, Springer, 2008

Dodge AM, Fitzer AF: When Good Doctors Get Sued: A Practical Guide for Physicians Involved in Malpractice Lawsuits. Olalla, WA, Dodge & Associates, 2006

Friedberg FJ: Surviving Your Deposition: A Complete Guide to Help You Prepare for Your Deposition. Atglen, PA, Schiffer Publishing, 2007

Gutheil TG: The presentation of forensic psychiatric evidence in court. Isr J Psychiatry Relat Sci 37:137–144, 2000

Gutheil TG: Deposition dos and don'ts: strategies for the expert witness. Psychiatr Clin North Am (in press)

Gutheil TG, Dattilio FM: Practical Approaches to Forensic Mental Health Testimony. Baltimore, MD, Lippincott, Williams & Wilkins, 2007

McCarthy ED: The Malpractice Cure: How to Avoid the Legal Mistakes That Doctors Make. New York, Kaplan, 2009

MD Mentor: Litigation stress. Available at: http://www.mdmentor.com/category/litigation-stress.

Physician Litigation Stress Resource Center Web site. Available at: http://www.physicianlitigationstress.org.

Simon RI, Sadoff RL: Psychiatric Malpractice: Cases and Comments for Clinicians. Washington, DC, American Psychiatric Press, 1992

Sloan FA, Chepke LM: Medical Malpractice. Boston, MA, MIT Press, 2010

Small DI: Preparing Witnesses: A Practical Guide for Lawyers and Their Clients, 2nd Edition. Chicago, IL, American Bar Association, 2004

Williams AG: Physician, Protect Thyself: 7 Simple Ways Not to Get Sued for Medical Malpractice. Pensacola, FL, Margol Publishing, 2007

Index

*Page numbers printed in **boldface** type refer to tables or figures.*